Pocket Guide to
Fetal Monitoring

Pocket Guide
to Fetal Monitoring

Susan Martin Tucker, R.N., M.S.N., P.H.N.

Director of Nursing, Maternal-Child Health
Kaiser Permanente Medical Center
Panorama City, California

Second Edition

with 71 *illustrations*

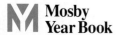

**Mosby
Year Book**

St. Louis Baltimore Boston Chicago London Philadelphia Sydney Toronto

Editor: Terry Van Schaik
Developmental Editor: Janet R. Livingston
Project Manager: Karen Edwards
Designer: Julie Taugner
Original Cover Art: Lynda Dümmel

Second Edition
Copyright © 1992 by Mosby–Year Book
A Mosby imprint of Mosby–Year Book, Inc.

Previous edition copyrighted 1988

Printed in the United States of America

Mosby–Year Book, Inc.
11830 Westline Industrial Drive
St. Louis, Missouri 63146

Library of Congress Cataloging-in-Publication Data
Tucker, Susan Martin
    Pocket guide to fetal monitoring / Susan Martin Tucker. —
    2nd ed. p. cm.
    Rev. ed of: Pocket nurse guide to fetal monitoring / Susan M.
Tucker. 1988.
    Includes bibliographical references and index.
    ISBN 0-8016-5232-4
    1. Fetal monitoring—Handbooks, manuals, etc.   2. Fetal heart
rate monitoring—Handbooks, manuals, etc.   3. Pediatric nursing—
Handbooks, manuals, etc.   I. Tucker, Susan Martin, Pocket nurse
guide to fetal monitoring.   II. Title.
    [DNLM: 1. Fetal monitoring—handbooks. 2. Fetal Monitoring-
nurses' instruction.   WQ 39 T894p]
RG628.T83   1992
618.3'207547—dc20
DNLM/DLC   91-46385
for Library of Congress   CIP

93 94 95 96 97 CL/DC/DC 9 8 7 6 5 4 3 2 1

Consultants

Cydney I. Afrait, C.N.M., M.S.N.
Assistant Clinical Professor
University of Rhode Island;
Clinical Teaching Associate
Brown University School of Medicine;
Certified Nurse Midwife
Women's and Infants Hospital
Providence, Rhode Island

Bonnie Flood Chez, R.N.C., M.S.N.
President
Nursing Education Resources, Inc.
Tampa, Florida

Bonnie J. Dattel, M.D.
Assistant Professor
Department of Obstetrics and Gynecology
   and Reproductive Sciences
University of California-San Francisco
San Francisco, California

Joan Drukker Dauphinee, R.N.C., M.S.
Director of Maternal Child Health
Magee-Women's Hospital
Pittsburgh, Pennsylvania

Lisa Milleman Garber, R.N.
Supervisor of Labor and Delivery
Kaiser Permanente Medical Center
Panorama City, California

Barbara J. Petree, R.N., M.A.
Nurse Educator and Staff Nurse
Stanford University Hospital
Palo Alto, California

Preface

Electronic fetal heart rate monitoring continues to be the most commonly used modality for the evaluation of fetal status during the intrapartum and antepartum periods. This fact is significant in light of studies demonstrating that auscultation of the fetal heart rate in low-risk patients is as effective as electronic monitoring. Efforts to control the cost of health care often preclude the ability of an institution to provide the necessary ratios of nurses to patients to perform periodic auscultation, and, as such, the use of electronic fetal monitoring serves to increase the productivity of the staff in the labor and delivery service.

The second edition of *Pocket Guide to Fetal Monitoring* provides both basic information for those who are new to electronic fetal heart rate monitoring and advanced information for the experienced practitioner. Chapter 1 introduces topical issues related to perinatal morbidity, mortality, and the incidence of cesarean section rates associated with electronic fetal monitoring. Chapter 2 explores the physiological basis for monitoring. In Chapter 3 auscultation of the fetal heart, instrumentation for electronic monitoring, and a section on troubleshooting the monitor are found along with a description of the advantages and limitations of each mode of monitoring. Uterine activity monitoring is described in Chapter 4 and is related to the use of stimulants and tocolytics. Baseline fetal heart rate patterns, periodic changes, unusual patterns, and fetal cardiac dysrhythmias are described in Chapters 5 and 6. In Chapter 7 reassuring fetal heart rate patterns are contrasted with those associated with fetal distress. In addition, other methods of assessment are described, including acoustic stimulation and acid-base monitoring. Interventions for fetal distress are delineated, as well as the use of amnioinfusion and tocolysis therapy. Antepartum monitoring, described in Chapter 8, contains sections on vibro-acoustic and nipple-stimulated contraction stress testing. In Chapter 9 the care of the patient on a fetal monitor is delineated. This chapter includes interventions based on the mode of monitoring, patient teaching guidelines, an equipment checklist, and guides for documentation and pattern interpretation. In Chapter 10 professional issues related to legal aspects, education, and competency are discussed, with reference to Appendix A, *Nursing Practice Competencies and Educational Guidelines: Antepartum Fetal Surveillance and Intrapartum Fetal Heart Monitoring,* by NAACOG. Standards of care are provided in Appendixes B, C, and D on oxytocin induction and augmentation of labor, the care of the patient in preterm labor and care of the patient in labor, and Appendix E includes patterns for practice interpretation.

The content of this pocket guide is designed for the practitioner who has a theoretical background in obstetrics. It can be used to assist in the management of patient care in the labor and delivery suite, the fetal intensive care unit, the LDR or LDRP (labor-delivery-recovery postpartum) unit, the antepartum inpatient unit, and the outpatient prenatal care setting. As an assessment technique used by physicians, nurse midwives, and nurses during the antepartum and intrapartum periods, electronic monitoring alone is not a basis for the nursing process. Nurses who wish to integrate the care of the electronically monitored patient with the nursing process are referred to the guideline for care of the patient in labor in Appendix D. The format of this book is designed to provide the user with readily retrievable instant information in an organized, logical sequence.

This book is offered in the hope that those who use it will be instrumental in enhancing the quality of life of the unborn and in promoting the quality of life of the newborn.

Susan Martin Tucker

Contents

Overview of Fetal Monitoring

1

The Problem

As we enter the most technically advanced period in perinatology, we are humbled by the fact that the United States has fallen to twentieth place among developed countries in the race to lower infant mortality. Some of our largest urban centers have infant mortality rates comparable to those in third world countries. The National Commission to Prevent Infant Mortality reports in "Troubling Trends: The Health of America's Next Generation" (February 1990) that several negative trends have been identified that prompt concern about maternal and infant care in the future. These include:

- Continuing high infant mortality with an infant death rate of 10.1 deaths per 1000 live births in 1987 and a decrease in the rate of decline from 4.7% per year in the 1970s to 2.7% per year in the 1980s
- No decline in the percentage of infants born at low birth weights, which is a major contributing factor to infant death and disability
- An increase in the infant mortality gap between white women and women of color
- An increase in the number of high-risk pregnancies associated with increases in crack use, AIDS, syphilis, and births to teenage mothers
- A higher percentage of births to women with inadequate prenatal care, including late care or no care at all

The Commission found that advances from expensive, high-tech perinatal medicine can no longer be relied on to significantly decrease infant mortality in the future. The final conclusion and recommendation of the report was that the answer to reversing the troubling trends of the 1980s lies in our nation's commitment to providing universal access to early maternity and pediatric care for all mothers and infants and in making the health and well-being of mothers and infants a national priority.

This information helps put into perspective the scope of the problem related to neonatal outcomes: that although they may be improved with the use of high-tech equipment during the perinatal and neonatal period, perfect outcomes cannot be guaranteed. Much of the present technology is taken for granted. There is now an array of biophysical, biochemical, and electronic techniques that monitor the fetus through the antepartum and intrapartum periods. It is easy to forget just how recent the developments have been to overcome the relative inaccessibility of the fetus to monitoring and evaluation.

Historical Overview

Fetal heart tones were first heard and described in the seventeenth century. Periodically, during the next 200 years, physicians described fetal heart tones or sounds and uterine souffle in medical journals. Then in 1917 Dr. David Hillis, an obstetrician at the Chicago Lying-In-Hospital, reported on the use of a head stethoscope, or fetoscope. The chief of staff at the same institution, Dr. J. B. DeLee, published a report regarding the use of a similar instrument to auscultate the fetal heart. Controversy developed when Dr. DeLee claimed to have had the idea before Dr. Hillis. The instrument that we know today as the fetoscope became known as the DeLee-Hillis stethoscope and has remained essentially unchanged in design and use.

The move to a higher level of technology was made in 1958 when Dr. Edward Hon of the Yale University School of Medicine published a report on continuous fetal electrocardiographic monitoring from the maternal abdomen. Dr. Caldeyro-Barcia of Uraguay and Dr. Hammacher of Germany reported their observations of fetal heart rate patterns associated with fetal distress in 1966 and 1967, respectively. In 1968 Dr. Ralph Benson et al. reported results of the collaborative study commissioned by the National Institute of Neurologic Diseases and Blindness. Some 24,863 deliveries were evaluated, and it was demonstrated that there was no correlation between the fetal heart rate as determined with fetoscope and neonatal condition, except in the most extreme circumstances. This was almost always fetal bradycardia auscultated before a terminal event. Ten years before Benson, Hon discovered the unreliability of counting fetal heart rate when he asked 15 obstetricians to count several rates from a tape recording of the fetal heart, and they found a wide divergence in counting.

As investigators throughout the world made similar observations of fetal heart rate decelerations and fluctuations from the baseline, a confusing array of terminology developed. At an international conference on fetal heart rate monitoring in December of 1971 in New Jersey, and later in March 1972 in Amsterdam, Doctors Hon, Caldeyro-Barcia, and their colleagues developed standard nomenclature for fetal heart rate monitoring. However, agreement on paper speed and universal scales was not reached and remained somewhat variable during the 1970s.

Since the first generation of commercially available fetal monitors in the late 1960s, technological advances have improved the quality and accuracy of the tracing. There is currently a proliferation of electronic fetal heart rate monitors on the market with some variations in capabilities; however, the basic components are the same.

There was widespread acceptance of electronic fetal heart rate monitoring in the 1970s with the majority of patients monitored during all or part of their labors. The hope for this technology was that it could prevent all or most cases of cerebral palsy. In addition, it had been hoped that electronic fetal monitoring would be more sensitive and accurate than intermittent auscultation in detecting fetal heart rate patterns that indicate fetal compromise.

Findings and Controversies

Several studies have indicated that there is either no change or perhaps a slight increase in the incidence of cerebral palsy in the past 25 years, during which time electronic fetal heart rate monitoring has been in use. It is difficult to determine if improved intrapartum care and appropriate intervention for abnormal heart rate patterns have contributed to a decrease in cerebral palsy, since increased survival rates for very low birth weight infants and improved neonatal care for asphyxiated infants has kept these numbers fairly constant.

Retrospective studies have correlated abnormal fetal heart rate patterns with low Apgar scores, fetal and neonatal acidosis, morbidity, and mortality. The infant mortality rate declined between 1970 and 1987 from 20.0 to 10.1 per 1000 live births. However, during this period the rate of cesarean sections increased because of a variety of factors, including changes in medical practice such as the performance of cesarean sections for breech presentations and the discontinuance of midforceps deliveries. It was suggested that there was a relationship between the increased cesarean section rate and the use of electronic fetal monitors. Governmental and consumer groups have been critical of this increase despite the fact that there has been an associated decrease in perinatal mortality. Cesarean section rates do vary among facilities because of demographic differences provided in the institution, but another variable is the ability of the staff to interpret patterns. Criticism by groups must be well taken in those facilities where personnel are not well trained and where there are no quality improvement activities such as a review of records by a multidisciplinary team of physicians and nurses for patients undergoing cesarean section for fetal distress based on the interpretation of the fetal monitor pattern.

The presumption that electronic fetal monitoring would be more sensitive and accurate than intermittent auscultation in detecting fetal heart rate patterns that indicate fetal compromise has not been supported by randomized prospective studies. In fact there are data that support the conclusion that intermittent auscultation is equivalent to continuous electronic fetal monitoring. It must be noted, however, that in the majority of these studies there was a 1:1 nurse/patient ratio. Because of the fluctuations in the numbers of patients in labor at any one point in time, it is very difficult, if not impossible, in some settings to provide this type of care from both a staffing and a cost factor standpoint.

Because of the wide acceptance and use of electronic fetal heart rate monitoring in today's busy obstetrical suites, it is doubtful that it will be abandoned in favor of auscultation, primarily because of the associated economic implications related to staffing. Auscultation, however, is a viable alternative to electronic monitoring and will be discussed in Chapter 3 for those who are able to monitor the fetus in this manner.

Physiological Basis for Monitoring

2

Electronic fetal monitoring (EFM) provides a technique for assessment of uterofetoplacental physiology and serves to indicate the adequacy of fetal oxygenation. Characteristic fetal heart rate (FHR) patterns are demonstrated as the result of hypoxic and nonhypoxic stresses or stimulation to the uterofetoplacental unit. Therefore it is important to have a basic understanding of the factors involved in fetal oxygenation, including uteroplacental circulation and physiology of FHR regulation.

Placenta and Intervillous Space

The placenta serves as a liaison between the fetal and maternal circulations (Figure 2-1). Oxygenated blood is delivered to the fetus through the umbilical vein. Deoxygenated blood returns to the placental chorionic villi through the two umbilical arteries. The chorionic villi are tiny vascular branches of the placenta that extend into the intervillous space. Maternal blood spurts upward from the uterine spiral arterioles and spreads laterally at random into the intervillous space, completely surrounding and bathing the villi (Figure 2-2). Although maternal and fetal blood are separated by a thin membrane and do not mix, several mechanisms occur whereby substances are exchanged across the placental membrane.

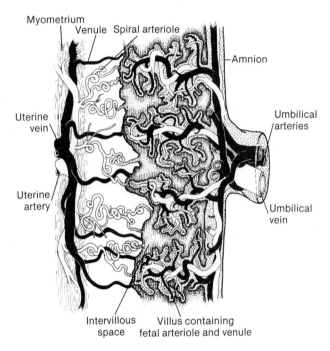

Figure 2-1
Schema of placenta.

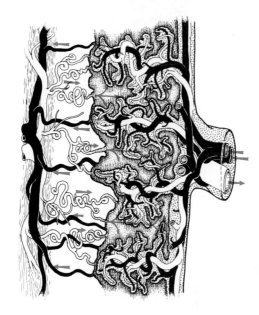

Figure 2-2
As maternal blood enters the intervillous space, it spurts upward from uterine spiral arterioles and spreads laterally at random.

Mechanisms occurring within intervillous space

The intervillous space then acts as a depot for the exchange of oxygen and nutrients and provides for the elimination of waste products. Together with the chorionic villi it functions as a fetal lung, gastrointestinal tract, kidney, skin (for heat exchange), infection barrier, and moderator of acid-base balance (Table 2-1).

At term some 700 to 800 ml of blood (10% to 15% of maternal cardiac output) perfuses the uterus each minute. Approximately 80% of this is within the intervillous space.

Table 2-1   Mechanisms occurring within intervillous space

Diffusion	Passage of substances from a region of higher concentration to one of lower concentration along a concentration gradient that is passive and requires no energy	Oxygen Carbon dioxide Small ions, (sodium, chloride) Lipids Fat-soluble vitamins Many drugs
Facilitated diffusion	Substances pass on the basis of a concentration gradient, probably a carrier molecule	Glucose Carbohydrates
Active transport	Passage of substances from one area to another against a concentration gradient; carrier molecules and energy are required	Amino acids Water-soluble vitamins Large ions, (calcium, iron, iodine)
Bulk flow	Transfer of substances by a hydrostatic or osmotic gradient	Water Dissolved electrolytes
Pinocytosis	Transfer of minute, engulfed particles across a cell	Immune globulins Serum proteins
Breaks or leakage	Small defects in the placental membrane allowing for passage of substances	Maternal or fetal blood cells and plasma (potentially resulting in isoimmunization)

Exchange of Gases

Transport and transfer of respiratory gases are of critical importance to fetal survival. Oxygen and carbon dioxide exchange are complex processes that depend on many physiological and biochemical factors. These include intervillous space blood flow, diffusing capacity of the placenta, placental area and vascularity, membrane permeability and thickness, oxygen tension of uterine and umbilical blood vessels, hemoglobin affinity and hemoglobin concentration of maternal and fetal blood, and fetal umbilical cord blood flow. Intervillous space blood flow has already been described. Further description of the other factors follows.

Diffusing capacity of placenta

The diffusing capacity of the placenta regulates the rate of oxygen transfer by a concentration gradient and the rate of blood flow. Oxygen diffuses from the maternal blood, which has a higher partial pressure, to the fetal blood, which has a lower partial pressure. Maternal and fetal blood flow rates can be altered by decreases in maternal blood pressure, as occurs with supine hypotension and following conduction anesthesia such as spinal, caudal, or epidural anesthesia; maternal exercise, uterine hypertonus or polysystole, decreased placental surface area (abruptio placenta or infarcts); or by increases in blood pressure, such as occurs with preeclampsia or vasoconstricting drugs.

Placental area

The larger and more vascular the placenta, the greater amount of substances that can be transferred between mother and fetus. Reduced placental area is associated with maternal hypertension, maternal diabetes, maternal vascular disease, fetal growth retardation, intrauterine infection, abruptio placentae, placenta previa, placental infarctions, and circumvallate placenta.

Oxygen tension

Oxygen tension in maternal arterial blood is determined by adequate pulmonary function. Diminished function resulting from maternal disease process or hypoventilation will decrease arterial oxygen tension (arterial Po_2). This can be remedied by adding inspired oxygen.

Oxygen transfer from maternal to fetal hemoglobin is regulated by the oxygen tension of the umbilical blood vessels. Generally, oxygen tension of the umbilical vessels is much lower than that of the maternal vessels (Figure 2-3). Some factors that compensate for this low fetal oxygen tension follow:
1. Increased fetal cardiac output (three to four times that of the resting adult per kilogram of body weight) based on heart rate
2. Increased oxygen-carrying capacity caused by high hemoglobin values (as compared with adult blood)

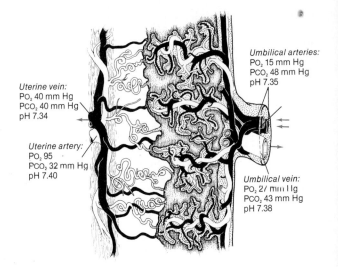

Figure 2-3
Maternal and fetal blood gas values.

3. Increased affinity of fetal blood for oxygen (as compared with adult blood) with a higher saturation of fetal hemoglobin at the same given Po_2 based on the fetal hemoglobin dissociation curve
4. Anatomical fetal shunts: ductus venosus, foramen ovale, and ductus arteriosis

Hemoglobin and oxygen affinity

Hemoglobin concentrations of maternal and fetal blood differ at term. Maternal hemoglobin is approximately 12 g/100 ml, in contrast with fetal hemoglobin, which is about 15 g/100 ml. Each gram of hemoglobin is capable of combining with 1.34 ml of oxygen. This increased oxygen-carrying capacity of fetal blood plus the high affinity of fetal blood for oxygen facilitate the transfer of oxygen from mother to fetus.

Umbilical blood flow

The mechanical force of a uterine contraction impedes intervillous space blood flow, exerts pressure directly on the fetus, and can occlude blood flow in both directions through the umbilical cord. Rapid fetal asphyxia with hypoxemia and acidosis can occur with entrapment and compression of the cord between fetal parts and the uterine wall. Transient cord compression occurs in about 40% of all labors, and the fetus is usually able to compensate in the intervals between contractions. However, in some labors in which the cord prolapses or is short, knotted, wrapped around fetal body parts, or where oligohydramnios is present, uncorrectable and prolonged variable deceleration of the fetal heart rate occurs. This is an obstetrical emergency, usually requiring immediate operative intervention, since fetal asphyxiation and death can occur. Amnioinfusion, the instillation of normal saline through an intrauterine catheter (a discussion of which can be found in Chapter 7), can act as a buffer between fetal parts and the uterine wall and can relieve variable decelerations caused by cord compression.

Decreased Uterine Blood Flow

Uterine blood flow is determined by uterine arterial and venous pressure and uterine vascular resistance. Some causes of decreased uterine blood flow follow.

Maternal position

A decrease in blood flow to the uterus can occur when the mother is in the dorsal recumbent position. The gravid uterus lies on the mother's vertebral column, exerting pressure on the great vessels, particularly the inferior vena cava. This pressure can compress this vessel, decreasing the volume of blood returning to the heart and producing a decrease in maternal cardiac output, hypotension, and a decrease in uterine blood flow. This mechanism is called *supine hypotension syndrome*.

Exercise

Fetal tachycardia that occurs after maternal exercise is thought to be due to a transitory period of reduced fetal oxygenation. Although maternal exercise diverts blood to the muscle groups and away from the uterus, there is no evidence that exercise is harmful when there is normal uteroplacental function.

Uterine contractions

Uterine contractions cause a decrease in the rate of perfusion of maternal blood through the intervillous space. Angiographic studies demonstrating this have shown impaired filling of the lobules with contrast medium during uterine contractions. In addition, fetal arterial blood oxygen tension decreases following the onset of each uterine contraction. The fetus, in most gestations, seems well able to compensate for these relatively minor stresses. However, in high-risk pregnancies in which the margin of fetal reserve is abnormally low, uterine contractions can cause some degree of hypoxia and commensurate decreases in the fetal heart rate, known as late decelerations. Recognition and treatment of late decelerations are described in Chapter 6.

To avoid compounding these stresses, it is important that the uterus relax adequately between contractions, that contractions not be excessively long, and that the tonus not rise. Intrauterine pressure between contractions—sometimes called *resting tone*—ranges from 5 to 15 mm Hg, with the average pressure between 8 and 12 mm Hg. During contractions intrauterine pressure ranges from 30 to more than 80 mm Hg, with an intensity of 50 to more than 100 mm Hg at the peak of the contraction. Angiographic studies show a cessation of maternal blood flow to the intervillous space with intrauterine pressures of 50 to 60 mm Hg during normal labor contractions.

It is thought that the fetus receives most of the oxygen and nutrients during the contraction and eliminates most of the carbon dioxide (CO_2) between contractions, and thus a healthy fetus with a normal placenta subjected to frequent contractions with inadequate uterine relaxation can become hypoxic and acidotic.

Uterine hypertonus

Uterine hypertonus—excessively high intrauterine pressure—can also cause the fetus to experience stress. Uterine hypertonus may occur spontaneously in some patients, particularly in those with a very distended uterus, as a result of hydramnios, multiple gestation, or macrosomia. Most frequently it occurs by uterine overstimulation with oxytocin. In some sensitive patients oxytocin produces tetanic contractions, characterized by high intrauterine pressure with absence of relaxation for a prolonged period. Abruptio placentae may also cause uterine hypertonus as a result of irritation of the myometrium from extravasated blood. In preeclampsia uterine resting tone is elevated because of vasoconstriction and decreased uterine blood flow. In addition, the following factors can interfere with placental perfusion and jeopardize the fetus:

1. Contractions lasting longer than 90 seconds
2. Relaxation between contractions that are less than 30 seconds
3. Inadequate decrease in intrauterine pressure between contractions

Surface area of placenta

The potential for fetal hypoxia is increased with any reduction in the placental surface area. Abruptio placentae is a clear example of this. Reduced placental area exposes the fetus to uteroplacental insufficiency and is associated with infarcts (as in hypertensive or prolonged pregnancies), maternal vascular disease, maternal diabetes, intrauterine infection, placenta previa, or circumvallate placenta.

Conduction anesthesia

Maternal hypotension caused by sympathetic blockade occurring with conduction anesthetics reduces blood flow in the intervillous space. Restoration of uterine blood flow is usually achieved by positional changes and expansion of maternal blood volume. Pressor agents, such as ephedrine, may also be required to restore maternal blood pressure.

Hypertension

Whether maternal hypertension is essential or pregnancy-induced, there is an increase in vascular resistance, resulting in a decrease in uterine blood flow.

Physiology of Fetal Heart Rate Regulation

The average fetal heart rate at term is 140 beats per minute (bpm). The normal range is 120 to 160 bpm. Earlier in gestation the fetal heart rate is much higher, with the average being ap-

Table 2-2   Regulatory control of fetal heart rate

Factors Regulating Fetal Heart Rate	Location
Parasympathetic division of autonomic nervous system	Vagus nerve fibers supply sinoatrial (SA) and atrioventricular (AV) node
Sympathetic division of autonomic nervous system	Nerves widely distributed in myocardium
Baroceptors	Stretch receptors in aortic arch and carotid sinus at the junction of the internal and external carotid arteries
Chemoceptors	Peripheral—in carotid and aortic bodies
	Central—in medulla oblongata
Central nervous system	Cerebral cortex
	Hypothalamus
	Medulla oblongata
Hormonal regulation	Adrenal medulla

Action	Effect
Stimulation causes release of acetylcholine at myoneural synapse	Decreases heart rate Maintains beat-to-beat variability
Stimulation causes release of norepinephrine at synapse	Increases FHR Increases strength of myocardial contraction Increases cardiac output
Responds to increase in blood pressure by stimulating stretch receptors to send impulses via vagus or glossopharyngeal nerve to midbrain producing vagal response and slowing heart activity	Decreases FHR Decreases blood pressure Decreases cardiac output
Responds to a marked peripheral decrease in O_2 and increase in CO_2	Produces bradycardia sometimes with increased variability
Central chemoceptors respond to decreases in O_2 tension and increases in CO_2 tension in blood and/or cerebrospinal fluid	Produces tachycardia and increase in blood pressure with decrease in variability
Responds to fetal movement	Increases variability
Responds to fetal sleep	Decreases variability
Regulates and coordinates autonomic activities (sympathetic and parasympathetic)	
Mediates cardiac and vasomotor reflex center by controlling heart action and blood vessel diameter	Maintains balance between cardioacceleration and cardiodeceleration
Releases epinephrine and norepinephrine with severe fetal hypoxia producing sympathetic response	Increases FHR Increases strength of myocardial contraction and blood pressure Increases cardiac output

Continued.

Table 2-2   Regulatory control of fetal heart rate—cont'd

Factors Regulating Fetal Heart Rate	Location
Hormonal regulation, cont'd	Adrenal cortex
	Vasopressin (plasma catecholamine)
Blood volume/capillary fluid shift	Fluid shift between capillaries and interstitial spaces
Intraplacental pressures	Intervillous space
Frank-Starling mechanism	Based on stretching of myocardium by increased inflow of venous blood into right atrium

Action	Effect
Low fetal blood pressure stimulates release of aldosterone, decreases sodium output, increases water retention, which increases circulating blood volume	Maintains homeostasis of blood volume
Produces vasoconstriction of nonvital vascular beds in the asphyxiated fetus	Distributes blood flow to maintain FHR and variability
Responds to elevated blood pressure by causing fluid to move out of capillaries and into interstitial spaces	Decreases blood volume and blood pressure
Responds to low blood pressure by causing fluid to move out of interstitial space into capillaries	Increases blood volume and blood pressure
Fluid shift between fetal and maternal blood is based on osmotic and blood pressure gradients; maternal blood pressure is about 100 mm Hg and fetal blood pressure about 55 mm Hg; therefore balance is probably maintained by some compensatory factor	Regulates blood volume and blood pressure
In the adult the myocardium is stretched by an increased inflow of blood, causing the heart to contract with greater force than before and pump out more blood; the adult then is able to increase cardiac output by increasing heart rate and stroke volume; this mechanism is not well-developed in the fetus	Cardiac output is dependent on heart rate in the fetus: $\downarrow$ FHR = $\downarrow$ cardiac output $\uparrow$ FHR = $\uparrow$ cardiac output

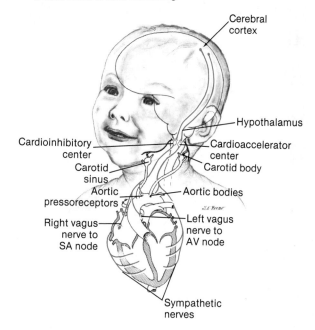

Figure 2-4
Schema of relation of control of FHR from central nervous system, parasympathetic and sympathetic divisions of autonomic nervous system, baroceptors, and chemoceptors.

proximately 160 bpm at 20 weeks' gestation. The rate progressively decreases as the fetus reaches term.

The heart rate is normally modulated by the sympathetic and parasympathetic nervous systems based on baroceptor and chemoceptor response (Figure 2-4). Regulatory control also depends on other factors, as described in Table 2-2.

Other factors that may influence the fetal heart rate are electrolyte imbalances such as hypokalemia (acceleration) and hypercalcemia (deceleration) and disturbances such as hyperthermia (acceleration) and hypothermia (deceleration).

Instrumentation for Fetal Heart Rate and Uterine Activity Monitoring

3

Overview

The goal of fetal heart rate monitoring is to detect signs that warn of potential adverse events in order to provide intervention in a timely manner. The fetal heart rate can be monitored by intermittent auscultation or by electronic means with an external or internal device. This chapter presents a description of devices that can be used to monitor the fetal heart rate and includes information on uterine activity monitoring, central display terminals, and telemetry. In addition, factors to be considered before purchasing an electronic monitor are provided.

Auscultation of Fetal Heart Rate
Description

In addition to the use of the electronic fetal monitor, auscultation of the fetal heart rate can be performed with a stethoscope, DeLee-Hillis fetoscope, or Doppler ultrasound device. If a *stethoscope* is used, the end should be turned so that the domed side of the stethoscope, rather than the flat side, is open to the connective tubing to the ear pieces. The domed side is then placed on the maternal abdomen. The *fetoscope* should be applied over the listener's head, since bone conduction amplifies the fetal heart sounds for counting. It is the ventricular fetal heart sounds that can be counted with the stethoscope and fetoscope.

The *Doppler ultrasound* device transmits ultra-high frequency sound waves to the moving interface of the fetal heart valves and deflects these back to the device, converting them into an electronic signal that can be counted.

Procedure	Rationale
1. Perform Leopold's maneuvers by palpating the maternal abdomen	1. To identify fetal presentation and position
2. Place the listening device over the area of maximum intensity and clarity of the fetal heart sounds, which is usually over the back of the fetus	2. To obtain the clearest and loudest sound, which is easier to count
3. Count the maternal radial pulse	3. To differentiate it from the fetal rate
4. Palpate the abdomen for the absence of uterine activity	4. To be able to count FHR between contractions
5. Count the fetal heart rate (FHR) for 30 to 60 seconds *between* contractions	5. To identify the baseline rate, which can only be assessed during the absence of uterine activity
6. Auscultate the FHR during a contraction and for 30 seconds after the end of the contraction	6. To identify the FHR during the contraction and as a response to the contraction
7. When there are distinct discrepancies in FHR during or between listening periods, auscultate for a longer period, both during, after, and between contractions	7. To identify changes from the baseline that indicate the need for another mode of FHR monitoring

Frequency of auscultation

Intermittent auscultation of the fetal heart rate should be performed at 15-minute intervals during the first stage of labor and at 5-minute intervals during the second stage of labor. In well-controlled research studies this frequency has been shown to be equivalent to continuous electronic monitoring in the assessment of the fetal condition. These studies did employ a ratio of one nurse to one patient, which should be employed if auscultation is used as the primary technique of fetal heart rate surveillance.

Auscultation of the FHR should occur *before* the administration of medications (including oxytocics and analgesics) and anesthetics, before periods of ambulation, and before artificial rupture of membranes. The FHR should be assessed immediately *following* rupture of membranes, changes in strength of uterine contraction (resting tone increase, sustained contraction, or tachysystole), vaginal examinations, changes in dosage of oxytocics, response to oxytocics, administration of medications (during peak action period), urinary catheterization, enema expulsion, period of ambulation, changes in dosage of anesthetic agents, and response to analgesics and anesthetics.

Documentation

Documentation of the fetal heart rate must be accompanied by other routine parameters that are assessed during labor, including uterine activity, maternal observations and assessment, and both maternal and fetal responses to interventions. It should be noted how long the heart rate was auscultated and whether this was before, during, and/or immediately after a uterine contraction. The rate, rhythm, and abrupt or gradual increases or decreases of the FHR during any part of this auscultated period should be described in relationship to the concurrent uterine activity. It is not appropriate to describe auscultated FHR using the descriptive terms associated with electronic fetal monitoring because the majority of the terms are visual descriptions of the patterns produced on the monitor tracing (e.g., early, late, and variable decelerations). However, terms that are numerically defined, such as bradycardia and tachycardia, can be used.

Interpretation

Reassuring fetal heart rate:

- FHR in the normal heart rate range without wide fluctuations from the average rate (which is obtained between contractions)

Nonreassuring fetal heart rate:

- An average FHR between contractions of less than 100 bpm
- A FHR of less than 100 bpm 30 seconds after a contraction

- Unexplained FHR of more than 160 bpm (tachycardia), especially if this occurs through three or more contractions in an at-risk patient

Management options of a nonreassuring fetal heart rate

- Continuous electronic fetal monitoring to validate FHR pattern. (This should be strongly considered for conditions that identify the fetus at risk for antepartum and/or intrapartum perinatal hypoxia or asphyxia. See the box below.)
- Fetal scalp sampling for pH
- Vibroacoustic stimulation with electronic monitoring to assess fetal response

---

High-Risk Conditions for Fetal Hypoxia/Asphyxia*

Postdates pregnancy
Pregnancy-induced hypertension or preeclampsia
Chronic hypertension
Diabetes mellitus
Intrauterine growth retardation
Preterm labor
Preterm rupture of membranes
Chronic renal disease
Active pulmonary disease
Cyanotic heart disease
Third trimester bleeding
Lupus or collagen vascular disease
Maternal anemia
Rh isoimmunization
Multiple gestation
Malpresentation
Hydramnios
Oligohydramnios
Meconium-stained amniotic fluid
Abnormal FHR on auscultation

---

*List is not all inclusive.

If nonreassuring patterns persist after attempts to correct them have been made, or if ancillary tests are not available or appropriate, then an expeditious delivery may be considered by the physician.

Advantages of auscultatory fetal heart rate monitoring

- Widely available and easy to use
- Noninvasive
- Inexpensive
- The sound of fetal heart tones confirms fetal life

Limitations

- May require maternal supine position, which could predispose to supine hypotension syndrome
- Does not provide a permanent, documented record
- The counting of FHR is intermittent
- Cannot assess FHR variability
- Nonreassuring events may occur during unmonitored periods
- Does not allow for early detection of nonreassuring patterns
- Can miss shallow, late decelerations that are associated with hypoxia

In summary, auscultatory fetal heart rate monitoring has been found to be effective if performed in a consistent manner by a nurse caring for one patient according to the the prescribed frequency. Because of the time and (nursing) labor-intensive nature of this method of monitoring, it may not always be an option in a busy unit that has the capability of continuous electronic fetal heart rate monitoring.

Electronic Fetal Monitoring

There are two modes of electronic monitoring. The external, or indirect, mode employs the use of external transducers placed on the maternal abdominal wall to assess FHR and uterine activity. The internal, or direct, mode uses a spiral electrode to assess the fetal electrocardiogram and the intrauterine or transcervical catheter to assess uterine activity and intrauterine pressure. A brief description contrasting the external and internal modes of monitoring (Figures 3-1 and 3-2) with a more detailed explanation of application and use follows.

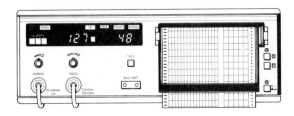

Figure 3-1
Electronic fetal monitor.

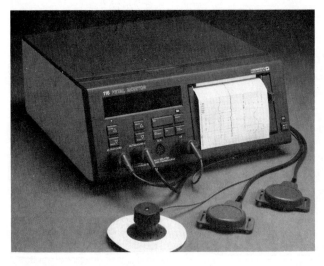

Figure 3-2
Fetal monitor with disposable adhesive baseplate on a beltless tocotransducer and two ultrasound transducers for the monitoring of twins.
(Courtesy Corometrics Medical Systems Inc., Wallingford, Conn.)

	External Mode (Indirect)	Internal Mode (Direct)
Fetal heart rate	Ultrasound (Doppler) transducer: High-frequency sound waves reflect mechanical action of fetal heart (easiest and most reliable external method to use during the antepartum and intrapartum periods) Abdominal electrodes: Fetal ECG is obtained when electrodes are properly positioned; it is used infrequently for antepartum monitoring because of ease and reliability of ultrasound transducer	Spiral electrode: Electrode converts fetal ECG as obtained from presenting part to FHR via cardiotachometer; this method can be used only when membranes are ruptured and the cervix is sufficiently dilated during the intrapartum period; electrode penetrates fetal presenting part 1.5 mm and must be securely attached to ensure a good signal
Uterine activity	Tocotransducer: This instrument monitors frequency and duration of contractions by means of a pressure-sensing device applied to the abdomen; it can be used during antepartum and intrapartum periods	Intrauterine catheter: This instrument monitors frequency, duration, and *intensity* of contractions; the catheter is compressed during contractions, placing pressure on the strain gauge mechanism and converts the pressure into mm Hg on the uterine activity panel of strip chart; it can be used only when membranes are ruptured and the cervix is sufficiently dilated during intrapartum period

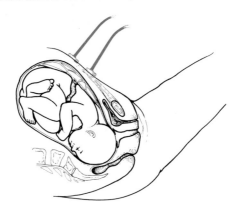

Figure 3-3
Placement of external transducers.

External mode of monitoring
Ultrasound transducer (Figure 3-3)
Description

Ultrasound, high-frequency sound waves, are transmitted by a transducer placed on the maternal abdomen. As the ultrasound strikes a moving interface—in this case the fetal heart and valves—a signal is directed back to the transducer, activating a tachometer. The FHR is printed out on the upper part of the strip chart, and a simultaneous indicator light on the monitor is observed with each heartbeat. This Doppler signal can be affected by changes in the position of the transducer or the fetus. Changes in the direction of the sound beam during uterine contractions may distort the tracing and mask periodic changes in the FHR. Because ultrasound reflects mechanical movement of the fetal heart, it cannot assess accurate short-term variability or beat-to-beat changes in the FHR. However, the monitors with autocorrelation capability very closely approximate accurate short-term variability. Newer monitors have dual ultrasound channels for the simultaneous monitoring of twins (Figures 3-4 and 3-5).

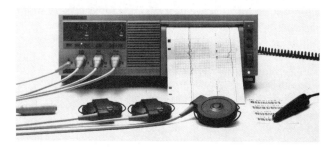

Figure 3-4
The HP M1350A fetal monitor from Hewlett-Packard
Company offers monitoring capabilities that include
dual-ultrasound twin monitoring, fetal-movement profile
(FMP), and a tocodynamometer transducer. Note barcode
reader that allows routine notations to be entered directly
on the tracing.
(Courtesy Hewlett-Packard Company, Andover, Mass.)

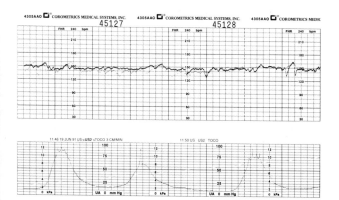

Figure 3-5
Dual ultrasonic heart rate monitoring strip demonstrates the
simultaneous, external monitoring of twins.
(Courtesy Corometrics Medical Systems Inc., Wallingford, Conn.)

The ultrasound transducer can be used to monitor FHR during both the antepartum and intrapartum periods. Correct placement of the ultrasound transducer depends on maternal cooperation and operator skill, since the transducer usually needs to be repositioned upon maternal position change. Excessive fetal movement can cause erratic operation of the FHR stylus. Very rapid changes in FHR, such as sudden variable decelerations, may not be followed completely by the ultrasound transducer.

A sequential format to assist the reader in a step-by-step approach follows:

Procedure	Rationale
1. Explain the procedure to the patient and her family	1. To allay anxiety
2. Gather necessary equipment: fetal monitor, ultrasound transducer, and either tocotransducer or intrauterine catheter apparatuses (to assess uterine activity), ultrasonic coupling gel, and abdominal belt	2. To ensure that all equipment is readily accessible
3. Position the patient in a semilateral position of comfort	3. To avoid supine hypotension syndrome
4. Insert the ultrasound transducer plug into the appropriate monitor connector labeled "ultrasound" or "cardio"	4. To connect cable plug to appropriate outlet
5. Plug the power cord into the electrical outlet; turn on the power, and gently touch the ultrasound diaphragm to elicit an equal audio response	5. To check for proper functioning of the transducer by simulating fetal heart sounds
6. Apply ultrasound coupling gel to the underside of the transducer placed on the maternal abdomen	6. To aid in the transmission of ultrasound waves (ECG paste frequently occludes this)

Procedure	Rationale
7. Place the transducer on the abdomen below the level of the umbilicus in a full-term pregnancy of cephalic presentation or above the level of the umbilicus in a full-term pregnancy of breech presentation	7. To search for the clearest signal, which is obtained by placing the transducer over the location of the fetal heart
8. Turn the audio-volume control knob while moving the transducer over the abdomen	8. To obtain the strongest fetal signal
9. Secure the ultrasound transducer with the abdominal belt or other fixation device.	9. To prevent displacement of transducer
10. Observe the indicator signal, which will flash simultaneously with each fetal heartbeat	10. To verify clarity of input and ensure correct placement of the transducer
11. Set the recorder at 3 cm/min paper speed and observe the FHR on the strip chart; obtain the baseline FHR *between* contractions or periodic changes	11. To ensure that paper feeds correctly and that recording is clear
12. Depress the test button for 10 seconds and make a notation of this on the tracing; ensure that the correct time is printed on the monitor strip (reset monitor clock as necessary) (Figure 3-6)	12. To ensure that the monitor prints out a predetermined number, usually 120 bpm on the corresponding line of the chart paper according to guidelines in manufacturer's operating manual
13. Periodically clean the transducer and maternal abdomen with a damp cloth to remove dried gel; reapply ultrasonic coupling gel and use talcum powder	13. To keep the skin dry and promote the patient's comfort

Procedure	Rationale

to dust under the abdominal belt if this is the fixation device

14. Reposition the transducer whenever the fetal signal becomes unclear, such as when the mother moves or when the fetus descends in the pelvis

14. To ensure a clear, interpretable tracing during fetal monitoring

15. When removing the ultrasound transducer, exercise caution so that it is not dropped or allowed to swing against any equipment; clean the transducer according to the procedure of the facility, or follow the directions in the manufacturer's operating manual

15. To protect the ultrasound crystals from damage

16. Loosely coil the cable and secure with a rubber band or place loosely coiled in a secure area

16. To prevent damage to the wires, which can occur with tight coiling, resulting in loss of, or an inadequate, fetal signal

17. Dispose of disposable abdominal belt; wash reusable belt according to the facility's procedure before the next patient's use

17. To ensure that disposable belt is not reused and that reusable belt is cleaned and ready for future use

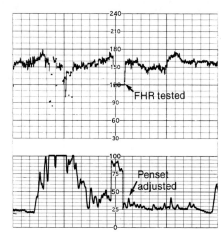

Figure 3-6
Testing of monitor: ultrasound and tocotransducer.

Advantages of the ultrasound transducer

- Noninvasive
- Easy to apply
- May be used during the antepartum period
- Does not require ruptured membranes or cervical dilatation
- No known hazards to mother or fetus

Limitations

- Requires patient cooperation in restricting some movement
- Requires repositioning with fetal or maternal position change that results in loss of signal
- Cannot accurately assess baseline FHR variability
- May double-count a slow FHR of less than 60 bpm (because of the inability to distinguish the first from the second heart sound so that they are both counted as equals)
- May half-count a tachydysrhythmia of more than 180 bpm (because of the inability to reset, which can result in the skipping or elimination of every other heartbeat)

- Maternal heart rate may be counted if the ultrasound is placed over the maternal arterial vessels, such as the aorta
- Obese patients may be difficult to monitor because of the distance between the transducer and the fetal heart

Abdominal ECG transducer
Description

The abdominal ECG transducer is capable of obtaining the FHR through the maternal abdominal wall. Most monitors use a system of blocking out the maternal ECG to prevent calculating the maternal heart rate. (Refer to the manufacturer's instruction manual for a description of this.) Long-term variability of the FHR can be assessed with the abdominal ECG transducer. Short-term variability cannot usually be assessed because of the circuitry, which when editing artifact, drops every sixth to eighth heartbeat, since these are coincident with the maternal heartbeat. This then serves to "clean up" the appearance of the FHR, resulting in a loss of a small amount of short-term variability information. The abdominal ECG transducer is best used in antepartum monitoring after 34 weeks' gestation and can be used for intrapartum monitoring, but generally works only if the patient is relaxed and lies still. A sequential format to assist the reader follows:

Procedure	Rationale
1. Explain the procedure to the patient and her family	1. To allay anxiety
2. Gather necessary equipment: fetal monitor abdominal electrodes, tocotransducer or intrauterine catheter (to assess uterine activity), electrode paste, alcohol swabs, and cable	2. To ensure that all equipment is readily available
3. Identify the fetal head and buttocks by palpating the maternal abdomen, using Leopold's maneuvers	3. To identify fetal presentation and position
4. Select the electrode application sites according to the manufacturer's operating manual; generally, one	4. To ensure that location of electrodes are in the best position to obtain a strong signal source

Procedure	Rationale
electrode will be positioned over the fetal head and one over the fetal buttocks; the third electrode is the reference and will be positioned below the umbilicus	
5. Prepare the skin sites with alcohol swabs by using a scrubbing motion; allow sites to dry	5. To remove all grease and promote adhesiveness of electrodes
6. If a built-in cleaner pad is affixed to the electrode protective cover, use it to gently abrade the skin at the selected electrode sites	6. To decrease electrical resistance of the maternal abdominal skin, which may obscure the low amplitude fetal ECG (FECG)
7. Rub in ECG paste	7. To promote ECG conduction
8. Remove excess paste	8. To promote electrode adhesion
9. Apply the pregelled disposable electrodes—one to the maternal skin site over the fetal head and the other just under the umbilicus	9. To obtain a strong fetal signal
10. Squeeze a thin bead of electrode paste around the rim of the suction electrode	10. To promote conduction of ECG
11. Apply the suction electrode to the maternal skin site over the fetal buttocks CAUTION: Do not leave a suction electrode in one location for more than 15 minutes	11. To prevent hematoma formation
12. Attach the lead wires to the electrodes according to manufacturer's operating	12. To ensure appropriate configuration of ECG

Procedure	Rationale
manual; generally, the lead wire with the white clip should be attached to the electrode over the fetal back (just below the maternal umbilicus); the lead wire with the black clip should be attached to the electrode over the fetal buttocks	
13. Insert the electrode cable plug into the appropriate monitor connector labeled "ECG" or "cardio"	13. To connect cable plug to appropriate outlet
14. Turn on the power and depress the edit button (if this is an option)	14. To reduce artifact and jitter
15. Observe the indicator light for a consistent flash with each fetal heartbeat	15. To verify a strong signal source
16. Set recorder at 3 cm/min paper speed and observe the FHR on the strip chart	16. To ensure that paper feeds correctly and that recording is clear
17. If the recording is clear, replace the suction cup with a disposable electrode; be sure to clean the electrode paste off the skin site and prepare the skin with alcohol, as described in steps 5 and 6.	17. To ensure adherence of electrode to skin
18. If a good recording cannot be obtained, conduct the following search procedure: a. Begin by moving the suction electrode over the fetal buttocks in a circular pattern from the original position to	18. To determine the best location for electrode placement

Procedure	Rationale
obtain the clearest fetal signal; replace the suction electrode with a disposable electrode once the best location has been determined	
b. If the signal continues to be unacceptable, perform the same procedure as in *a*, but replace other electrodes in sequence until a clear signal is obtained	
c. Should the signal continue to be unacceptable after repositioning the three electrodes, another method of monitoring FHR should be used	
19. If the monitor has the capability of displaying the maternal heart rate on the light-emitting diode (LED) and printing this out on the chart paper, a printout can be obtained by depressing the maternal heart rate button for as long as a record of the maternal heart rate is desired	19. To distinguish maternal from fetal heart rate
20. Observe the indicator light, which will flash simultaneously with each ECG complex	20. To verify a clear signal source
21. Depress the test button for 10 seconds and make a notation of this on the tracing; be certain that the monitor clock reflects the accurate time	21. To ensure that the monitor will print out a predetermined number, usually 120 or 150 bpm, on the corresponding line of the chart paper according to guidelines in the manufacturer's operating manual

It may be difficult or impossible to obtain an interpretable reading in the following situations: (1) oligohydramnios or hydramnios, (2) multiple gestation, (3) gestational age of less than 34 weeks (because of a low-voltage fetal signal), and (4) periods of maternal muscle activity and tension, such as the active phase of labor.

Advantages of the abdominal ECG transducer

- Noninvasive
- May be used during antepartum or early labor periods

Limitations

- Maternal movement and muscle activity may interfere with the tracing
- Data may be lost when maternal and fetal signals occur at the same moment
- Difficult to obtain a consistently clear tracing

Tocotransducer (tocodynamometer)
Description

The tocotransducer monitors uterine activity transabdominally by means of a pressure-sensing button that is depressed by uterine contractions or fetal movement. The uterine activity panel of the chart paper displays frequency and duration of contractions. Absolute intensity can be assessed only with the intrauterine catheter. The tocotransducer can be used to monitor uterine activity during both the antepartum and intrapartum periods.

A sequential format is provided to assist the reader.

Procedure	Rationale
1. Explain the procedure to the patient and her family	1. To allay anxiety
2. Gather the necessary equipment: fetal monitor, tocotransducer (tocodynamometer), and the equipment desired to monitor the FHR	2. To ensure that all equipment is readily accessible
3. Position the abdominal belt around the patient's upper abdomen, over the uterine	3. To avoid supine hypotension syndrome

Procedure	Rationale
fundus, and place her in a semilateral position of comfort	
4. Insert the tocotransducer plug into the appropriate monitor connector labeled "uterine activity," "toco," or "utero"	4. To connect cable plug to appropriate outlet
5. Place the transducer on the maternal abdomen over the fundus where there is the least amount of maternal tissue between the pressure-sensing button and the uterus, (where uterine contractions are best palpated)	5. To ensure that the fundus is as close as possible to the pressure-sensing button
6. Secure the tocotransducer with the abdominal belt	6. To prevent displacement of the transducer
7. Set the recorder at 3 cm/min paper speed and observe the strip chart	7. To ensure that the paper feeds correctly and that recording is clear
8. Adjust the sensitivity calibration device between contractions to print at the 20 or 25 mm Hg line on the chart paper (see Figure 3-6)	8. To prevent missing the very beginning or ending of the uterine contraction, which is necessary for FHR pattern interpretation.
9. Test the tocotransducer by applying slight pressure and observe the strip chart for a relative inflection of momentary increase from the "baseline"	9. To ensure that the transducer is pressure sensitive
10. Monitor the frequency and duration of the contractions and document them in the nurse's notes	10. The tocotransducer *cannot* measure intensity of contractions or resting tone between contractions, because the depression of the pressure-sensing button

Procedure	Rationale
	varies with the amount of maternal adipose tissue; therefore the information should not be relied on to assess need for analgesia in relation to strength (painfulness) of contractions as registered by the monitor
11. When monitoring is in progress, readjust the abdominal strap periodically, and massage any reddened skin areas; a small amount of powder can be applied under the belt	11. To promote comfort and maintain the proper position of the transducer
12. Palpate the fundus every 15 to 30 minutes; *do not* rely on "peak pressure" of contraction to determine need for analgesia	12. To assess relative pressure of contraction, because tocotransducer can relate only frequency and duration of contractions; it cannot assess intensity or resting tone
13. Reposition the transducer periodically and secure the abdominal belt snugly	13. To promote and ensure a good recording
14. When removing the tocotransducer, follow the procedure of the facility or follow the manufacturer's directions in the operating manual	14. To protect the surface of the transducer
15. Loosely coil the cable and secure with a rubber band, or place loosely coiled in a secure area	15. To prevent damage to the wires, which can occur with tight coiling
16. Dispose of disposable abdominal belt; wash reusable belt according to the facility's procedure before the next patient's use	16. To ensure that a disposable belt is not reused and that a reusable belt is cleaned and ready for future use

Advantages of the tocotransducer

- Noninvasive
- Does not require ruptured membranes or cervical dilatation
- Is easily applied
- May be used with telemetry

Limitations

- Information is limited to frequency and duration
- Cannot assess intensity of contractions
- Periodic repositioning of transducer may be necessary
- Limits patient's mobility
- May not get an interpretative tracing from an obese patient

Internal mode of monitoring (Figure 3-7)
Spiral Electrode
Description

The spiral electrode monitors the fetal ECG from the presenting part. It can be applied only after the membranes are ruptured, when the cervix is 2 to 3 cm or more dilated, and when the presenting part is accessible and identifiable. Therefore the spiral electrode can be used only during the intrapartum period. Use of the spiral electrode is contraindicated in patients suspected of

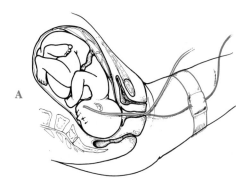

Figure 3-7
A, Diagrammatic representation of internal mode of monitoring with intrauterine catheter and spiral electrode in place.

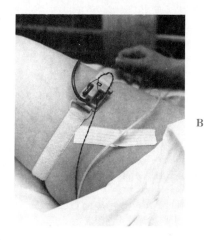

B

Figure 3-7, cont'd
B, Spiral electrode connected to leg plate and intrauterine catheter secured to patient's thigh.

having active herpes or group B streptococcus or when there is undiagnosed vaginal bleeding (rule out placenta previa).

A sequential format provided to assist the reader follows:

Procedure	Rationale
1. Explain the procedure to the patient and her family	1. To allay anxiety
2. Gather necessary equipment: fetal monitor, disposable spiral electrode, leg plate with cable, leg plate strap, and electrode paste	2. To ensure that all equipment is readily accessible
3. Position the leg plate strap around the woman's thigh, securing the leg plate to the thigh; gently lift the leg plate and apply electrode paste to the underside	3. To ensure transmission of electrical signal

Procedure	Rationale
4. Insert the cable into the appropriate monitor connector labeled "ECG" or "cardio"	4. To connect cable plug to appropriate outlet
5. Assist the physician or nurse in performing a sterile vaginal examination in order to apply the spiral electrode a. Insert the entire apparatus through the vagina and cervix against the fetal presenting part b. Rotate the inner tube clockwise one full turn c. Remove and discard the outer drive tube	5. The electrode must be securely attached to ensure a good signal; the fetal face, fontanels, and genitals are avoided, and the electrode penetrates the skin of the presenting part 1.5 mm
6. Attach the wires to the posts on the leg plate	6. To provide proper polarity for ECG tracing
7. Turn on the power and observe the indicator light	7. To allow time for the monitor to warm
8. Set the recorder at 3 cm/min paper speed, and observe the FHR on the strip chart	8. To ensure that the paper feeds correctly and that the recording is clear
9. Depress the test button for 10 seconds and make a notation of this on the strip chart; ensure that the monitor clock reflects the accurate time	9. To ensure that the monitor prints out a predetermined number (usually 120 or 150 bpm) on the corresponding line of the chart paper according to the manufacturer's guidelines in the operating manual
10. During monitoring the leg plate is checked periodically, and electrode paste is reapplied as needed NOTE: The spiral/electrode must be moist in vaginal secretions or signal transmission may be impaired	10. To ensure transmission of the signal

Procedure	Rationale
11. When removing the spiral electrode, turn 1½ turns counterclockwise or until it is free from the fetal presenting part; do not pull the electrode from the fetal skin; disconnect the electrode from the leg plate NOTE: The electrode should be removed just before cesarean delivery and should not be left attached and brought up through the uterine incision	11. To ensure that the electrode is removed in the same manner that it is applied; pulling the electrode straight out results in unnecessary trauma to the fetal skin, produces an observable wound, and predisposes the site to infection
12. Remove the leg strap and dispose of it, if it is disposable, or wash if it is reusable	12. To ensure that the disposable belt is not reused and that the reusable belt is cleaned and ready for future use
13. Clean the leg plate according to the facility's procedure, or follow the manufacturer's directions in the operating manual	13. To remove any dried ECG paste
14. Loosely coil the cable and secure with a rubber band, or place loosely coiled in a secure area	14. To prevent damage to the wires, which can occur with tight coiling, resulting in loss of, or an inadequate, fetal signal
15. Clean the fetal insertion site with a povidone-iodine swab unless otherwise directed by hospital policy or procedure	15. To prevent infection

Advantages of the spiral electrode

- Can assess variability
- Positional changes do not affect quality of tracing
- Can accurately display fetal cardiac dysrhythmias
- Accurately displays FHR between 30 and 240 bpm

Limitations

- Membranes must be ruptured
- Cervix must be dilated at least 2 cm
- Presenting part must be accessible
- May record maternal heart rate (with fetal demise)

Intrauterine (transcervical) catheter
Description

The intrauterine catheter monitors contraction frequency, duration, intensity, and resting tone. A small catheter is introduced vaginally (transcervically) into the uterus after the cervix is dilated 2 to 3 cm and the fetal membranes have been ruptured. The catheter is compressed during uterine contractions, placing pressure on a strain gauge, or pressure transducer. The pressure is then reflected on the strip chart in the form of mm Hg pressure.

Some newer internal pressure catheters have the pressure sensing device within the catheter tip. These do not require the instillation of sterile water for use. Some of these newer catheters are provided with a double lumen to allow simultaneous amniofusion and uterine activity monitoring.

Procedure	Rationale
1. Explain the procedure to the patient and her family	1. To allay anxiety
2. Gather necessary equipment: fetal monitor, disposable intrauterine kit, sterile gloves, and other equipment to perform a sterile vaginal examination	2. To ensure that all equipment is readily accessible
3. Insert the reusable cable into the appropriate monitor connector labeled "uterine activity," "toco," or "utero"	3. To activate the pressure transducer
4. Before inserting a "fluid-filled catheter" fill the catheter with 5 ml sterile water, leaving the syringe attached to the catheter; maintain sterility of the	4. To ensure that the catheter is patent and fluid-filled before insertion; to maintain aseptic technique

Procedure	Rationale

maternal end of the catheter

5. Prepare the patient for a sterile vaginal examination; the examining fingers are placed just inside the cervix

5. To maintain aseptic technique and to identify the location for catheter insertion

6. Insert the sterile catheter within the catheter guide no more than 2 cm inside the cervix

6. The guide is made of a very hard plastic that can cause trauma if inserted farther than necessary

7. Advance the catheter according to the insertion depth indicator or until the blue or black mark on it reaches the vaginal introitus

7. To ensure that enough of the catheter is inside the uterus

8. Slide the catheter guide away from the introitus and remove it from the opposite end, (or after cleaning the guide, tape it securely over the top or across the side of the monitor)

8. To prevent the guide from sliding toward the introitus

9. Tape the catheter securely to the patient's leg

9. To ensure patient mobility without fear of dislodging the catheter

10. Connect the intrauterine catheter transducer to the cable or connect the fluid-filled catheter to the strain gauge apparatus (pressure transducer) via the three-way stopcock.

10. To ensure appropriate location of strain gauge in relation to the uterus

Perform the following procedures only for fluid-filled catheters:

a. Test or calibrate the strain gauge according to the manufacturer's instructions

a. To validate that uterine activity information is correct

Procedure	Rationale
b. Maintaining the stopcock "Off" to the strain gauge, flush the catheter with 5 ml sterile water	b. To ensure that the catheter is patent and completely filled with fluid
c. Rotate the stopcock lever so that the "Off" position points to the catheter	c. To exclude pressure to the strain gauge
d. Release the pressure valve on the strain gauge and inject water from the syringe through the stopcock and gauge until all air bubbles are removed	d. To ensure that the strain gauge is completely filled with fluid
e. Release the pressure relief valve and then remove the syringe from the stopcock, maintaining its sterility	e. To open the system to atmospheric pressure
f. Turn on the power and press the record button; observe the tracing, which should print on the zero line of the uterine activity section of the chart paper; turn the pressure knob to ensure that the pen reads just at the zero line of the chart paper; *(do not turn it to go below zero)*	f. To verify that the tracing prints out on the zero line in the absence of pressure
g. Depress the test button for 10 seconds and make a notation of this on the tracing; the monitor will print a predetermined number, usually at the 50 mm	g. To ensure that the monitor traces on the appropriate line; this validates the accuracy of subsequent internal pressure monitoring

Procedure	Rationale
Hg line of the chart paper, according to the manufacturer's operating manual; if it does not read 50 mm Hg, adjust the pressure knob to ensure that the pen points at the zero line of the chart paper and then test it again (Figure 3-8)	
h. Reattach the syringe to the stopcock; rotate the stopcock lever so that the "Off" position is pointing to the syringe; the uterine pressure system is now ready for monitoring	h. The solid column of water places pressure on the diaphragm of the strain gauge when it is compressed by uterine contractions; this results in an inflection on the uterine activity section of the strip chart in mm Hg
i. When monitoring is in progress:	
(1) Flush the intrauterine catheter with sterile water every 2 hours or as necessary (The use of solutions other than sterile water can occlude and corrode the system)	(1) To remove any vernix caseosa or air bubbles that may have entered the catheter and can invalidate the pressure reading
(2) Check the proper functioning of the catheter when necessary by tapping the catheter, asking the patient to cough, or applying fundal pressure while observing the chart	(2) To ensure inflection on the chart paper

Procedure	Rationale
11. Zero the catheter and test according to the manufacturer's directions	11. To ensure that the monitor traces on the appropriate line; this validates the accuracy of subsequent internal pressure monitoring
12. Apply gentle traction to remove catheter and dispose of catheter appropriately	12. To ensure that disposable equipment is not reused

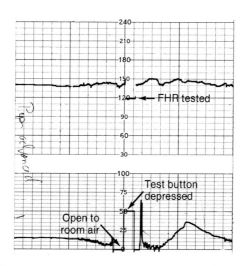

Figure 3-8
FHR and uterine activity tested for internal mode of monitoring.

Advantages of the intrauterine catheter

- Less confining and more comfortable than external mode of uterine activity monitoring
- Only accurate measure of uterine activity (e.g., frequency, duration, intensity, and resting tone)
- May be used with telemetry
- Records accurately regardless of maternal position

Limitations

- Membranes must be ruptured and cervix sufficiently dilated (e.g., 2 to 3 cm)
- Improper insertion can cause maternal trauma
- Increased risk of infection

Troubleshooting the monitor

The electronic fetal monitor is a useful tool to assess fetal well-being. As with any electronic device, problems may occur that can often be overcome. The following section suggests actions for identified problems.

Problem	Action
Power	■ Check power cord at wall and back of monitor
	■ Push in both ends of cord to ensure a tight fit (it may appear intact, although it is not)
Sixty-cycle interference	■ Check FHR by auscultation
	■ If there is improper grounding at the outlet, plug, or in machine, change to another electrical outlet, switch cords, or change electrode wires (on ground cable)
	■ Change electrode or monitor
	■ Reverse polarity switch on some old monitors

Problem	Action
Ultrasound *Half or double rate*	▪ Check with fetoscope, stethoscope, or Doppler
	▪ Check maternal pulse to rule out maternal signal
	▪ Consider applying spiral electrode, or call physician to apply electrode if membranes are intact and bradycardia is present
	▪ Add coupling gel and recheck
	▪ Move transducer to search for a better signal
Intermittent ultrasound signal	▪ Check ultrasound transducer: hold transducer by cord, allow transducer to hang, turn up volume, swing ultrasound transducer in the air; if static is heard, replace transducer; apply label to broken transducer for repair or replacement
	▪ Check cable insertion site for a tight fit
Intermittent or no signal	▪ Check gel on transducer; it may be dry. (When dry, sound waves do not penetrate the skin); reapply gel; Move transducer if fetus is out of range
Autocorrelation limitations	▪ Compares new data to last several beats; at times can exclude data from the comparison or can produce a false signal in the absence of fetal cardiac motion by enhancing signal-to-noise levels

Problem	Action
Direct FHR monitoring with spiral electrode	
Intermittent signal (individual dots on monitor strip or no signal)	■ Do vaginal exam; check electrode placement; if loose, replace electrode
	■ Check that reference electrode is in vaginal secretions. (Instill fluid if necessary)
	■ Check ground cable on leg for adherence to skin
	■ If still no signal, remove red wire from ground cable, replace with disposable electrode and reference electrode wire
Signal and recording with stillborn (maternal signal is conducted through the stillborn infant)	■ Check maternal pulse (radial)
	■ Check with doptone and suggest ultrasound to check for heart motion
Uterine activity *Tocodynamometer (toco)*	
■ No recording	■ Readjust toco on patient
■ Numbers in high range	■ Turn down the setting to a lower number on toco channel; (if numbers cannot be turned down, toco needs repair); replace with another toco
Toco not picking up contractions	■ Palpate abdomen for best quality of contractions and reapply toco
	■ Place elastic belts tighter, or use another device to hold toco firmly against abdomen
	■ Consider using IUPC if patient is significantly obese

Problem	Action
Intrauterine pressure catheter (IUPC)	
Not recording	■ Recheck cable insertion
■ Resting tone (6 to 15 mm Hg)	■ Adjust level of strain gauge for fluid-filled catheters
	■ Flush fluid-filled catheter
	■ Recalibrate nonfluid-filled catheter
Not recording contractions	■ Check catheter markings at patient's introitus (catheter may have slipped out)
	■ Replace catheter if necessary
High resting tone	■ Higher resting tone may be noted for Pitocin (20 mm Hg) Twins (30 mm Hg) Amnionitis (30 to 40 mm Hg)
Other problems *Dysrhythmia*	
	■ Occurs in 5% of pregnancies
	■ Turn up volume (can dysrhythmia be heard?)
	■ Consult with other health professionals
	■ Check for variability, tachycardia, and bradycardia
	■ Perform fetal ECG
Errors caused by incorrect paper speed or monitor paper with different scale	■ Check annotation with paper speed; it should be 3 cm/min
	■ Check scale; it should be 30 to 240 bpm for FHR

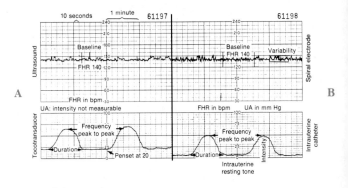

Figure 3-9

Display of FHR and uterine activity on monitor strip. **A,**
External mode: ultrasound and tocotransducer are the signal
sources. **B,** Internal mode: spiral electrode and intrauterine
catheter are the signal sources. Other significant information
is supplied.

Display of fetal heart rate and uterine activity (Figure 3-9)

FHR is recorded on the upper section of the chart paper, and
uterine activity is recorded on the lower section. The FHR is
printed on a vertical scale with a range of 30 to 240 bpm. The
horizontal scale is divided into 1-minute sections, which are sub-
divided by six sections representing 10 seconds each.

The lower section is used to record uterine activity. The vertical scale ranges from 0 to 100 mm Hg pressure and is accurate
in assessing intensity of contractions only when the intrauterine
catheter is used. The horizontal scale represents time as previously described. The lower section of the chart paper can be used
to assess frequency of contractions, usually measured from peak
to peak, (or from onset of one uterine contraction to the onset of
the next uterine contraction) and duration of contractions. Because the inflections of uterine activity, which are noted on the
chart paper and assessed with the tocotransducer, are dependent
on the thickness of maternal adipose tissue and tocotransducer
placement over the maternal uterine fundus, it must be remem-
bered that the intensity of uterine contractions cannot be assessed
by use of the external mode of monitoring.

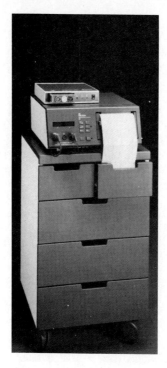

Figure 3-10
Telemetry unit on top of fetal monitor.
(Courtesy Corometrics Medical Systems, Inc., Wallingford, Conn.)

Telemetry

Remote internal or external FHR monitoring via radio wave telemetry (Figure 3-10) helps patients to remain ambulatory without the loss of continuous monitoring data. The patient may feel
less confined, more relaxed, and more content if she can walk
around. The transducer is worn by the patient by means of a
shoulder strap or other device (Figure 3-11). Heart rate and uterine activity signals are continuously transmitted to a receiver that
is connected to the fetal monitor. The monitor then processes the
data, displays, and prints the heart rate and uterine activity on the
strip chart.

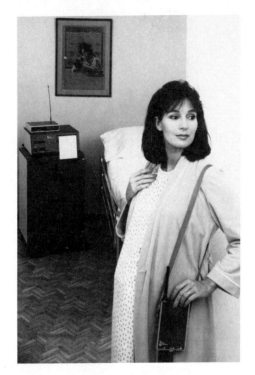

Figure 3-11
Ambulatory patient being monitored with telemetry unit.
(Courtesy Corometrics Medical Systems, Inc., Wallingford, Conn.)

In addition to the benefits of freedom of movement during labor and continuous monitoring during transport within the labor suite or to the delivery room, telemetry has been applied in the outpatient setting for patients instructed to remain at rest in their own homes. Data from the transmitter can be sent via modem to the receiver unit, which is connected to a printer, producing a hard copy of the FHR strip chart. This transmission of information from the patient to the receiver unit allows the clinician to determine the patient's status. Based on the data received, the patient's tocolytic needs may be adjusted, and consultation can be made with a referral center by the clinician to receive an expert's interpretation of the data.

Central display (Figure 3-12)

Central monitor display at the nurses' station provides an opportunity to view tracings from several patients at the same time. In addition, single screen display of several patients can be accessed from remote locations including the patient's bedside, staff locker room or lounge areas, or a physician's office. This can provide the staff with instant access to the patient's monitor pattern from any location and is especially important when the nurse cannot be in constant attendance. Some systems include the capability of data entry in the form of detailed notes about results of examinations, cervical dilatation, fetal station, administration of

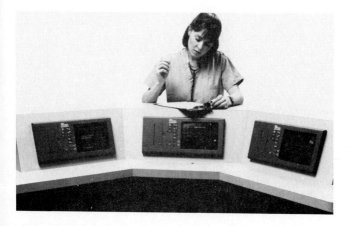

Figure 3-12
Central display unit with capability of displaying individual patient trends or automatically scanning all or a portion of up to 20 bedside monitors.
(Courtesy Corometrics Medical Systems, Inc., Wallingford, Conn.)

drugs, patient's position, and vital signs, all related to time. Reports may be generated with the integration of an optional printer linked to the display, which can contain complete patient information, history, and a graphic printout of the labor curve progression, providing a single and comprehensive document.

Some central display systems can provide additional information, including the following:

1. A system status screen provides an instant overview of several beds on the system and indicates any alerts by room number. In addition, it can identify the signal source of any of the patients on the system.

2. A trend screen, which can provide the most recent past few minutes of heart rate and uterine activity data on any one patient, with immediate warning of critical conditions relating to any patient in the system.

3. An alert screen, which provides an immediate summary of the trend analysis on any patient. The data can be made available to the staff before, during, and after an alert.

Archival and retrieval

Traditional long-term storage of fetal monitoring strips has been problematic for most medical record units in terms of time and space. Microfiche records of the strip chart are less bulky to store but still take time to log, sort, and file in the medical record. An alternative to this is the capability of new central monitoring systems that store patient information and data from the monitors, including direct intrapartum and antepartum recordings. The data are stored by the central computer on hard drives or floppy disks. Some systems with optical disk storage hold approximately 28,000 hours of monitor data, which is enough for about 3000 patients. The ability to record, store, retrieve, and reproduce the tracing is a significant advance in the archiving and retrieval of fetal monitoring data.

Data input devices

Data input devices are now an option with some electronic fetal monitors and monitoring systems. Some of the options include use of a barcode reader, key pads for data entry (Figure 3-13), and standard typewriter keyboards. The input is subsequently printed on the strip chart (Figure 3-14). The use of these options can promote accurate documentation and help to eliminate the

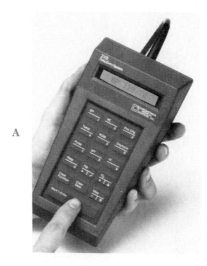

A

B

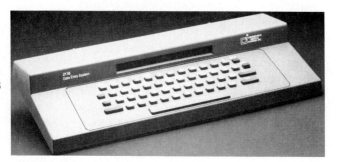

Figure 3-13
A, Data entry keypad helps to eliminate the need for handwritten annotations and can be used at the patient's bedside. **B,** The data entry keyboard is programmed to print obstetrical parameters.
(Courtesy Corometrics Medical Systems, Inc., Wallingford, Conn.)

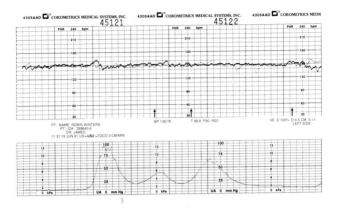

Figure 3-14
Tracing demonstrates pertinent data that has been entered
via a data input device.
(Courtesy Corometrics Medical Systems, Inc., Wallingford, Conn.)

need for handwritten annotations, which are sometimes illegible.
In addition, some information may be entered on the strip chart
automatically, including time (every 10 minutes), date, chart
speed, monitoring, and baseline pressure off scale.

Artifact detection

Fetal monitors have built-in artifact rejection systems, which are
always in operation when using the external mode of FHR monitoring. Logic circuitry rejects data when there is a greater variation than is expected between successive fetal heartbeats. If there
are repetitive variations by more than the accepted amount, the
older generation monitors may switch from a hold mode to a
nonrecord mode (exhibited by penlift or no heat to the stylus).
The recorder resumes recording when the variation between successive beats falls within the predetermined parameters. The
newer monitors continue to print regardless of the extent of the
excursion of the fetal heart rate.

During internal monitoring, artifact is rare, and the logic system will miss only those changes that exceed the predetermined
limits of the system. If there is an accessible switch to select a
logic or no-logic mode, it is preferable to have the monitor in the
no-logic mode when using the internal mode (spiral electrode) in
order to detect fetal arrhythmias. When recording internally, the

logic-on should be used only when there is true artifact, such as with poor signal-to-noise ratio (caused by extraneous electrical noise), or when there is a large maternal R wave that is counted on an intermittent basis. This can usually be determined by printing out the fetal ECG.

Considerations before monitor purchase

Various monitors are available, and generally they have the same capabilities. In considering a monitor for purchase, however, it is prudent to use the desired model on a trial basis and to consult with people who have used the type of equipment being considered. The following items should also be considered:

1. Accuracy of data output
2. Ease of use
3. Reliability for continuous functioning with minimum down/repair time
4. Repair history from other facilities using the same monitor, (turnaround time for service)
5. Cost of monitor and other expendable supplies (e.g., paper, abdominal belts)
6. Legible display and function labels
7. Complexity of paper refill procedure
8. Training time needed for users
9. Fragility of ultrasound transducer, cable, and connectors
10. History and stability of company and frequency of changing models
11. Expected life of the equipment
12. Interchangeability of transducers from one model to the next within the same company (to avoid the possibility of built-in obsolescence)

Uterine Activity Monitoring

4

One of the benefits of electronic FHR monitoring is the data provided about uterine activity. Frequency and duration of uterine contractions can be determined by manual palpation, but the intensity of the contractions cannot be measured in this manner. In addition to quantifying intensity of contractions via the intrauterine catheter, the monitor provides a permanent record of uterine activity.

Uterine activity is monitored on the lower section of the chart panel. Each major vertical division represents 25 mm Hg pressure, with the smaller lines representing 5 mm Hg. There are major differences between the external mode of monitoring and the internal mode in terms of obtainable uterine activity data. The following list contrasts these two modes of monitoring:

	External Mode	Internal Mode
SIGNAL SOURCE	Tocotransducer (tocodynamometer)	Intrauterine (transcervical) catheter
DATA	1. Frequency of contractions (measured from peak to peak or from the onset of one contraction to the onset of the next contraction)	1. Frequency of contractions (measured from peak to peak or from the onset of one contraction to the onset of the next contraction)
	2. Duration of contractions (from beginning to end)	2. Duration of contractions (from beginning to end)

External Mode	Internal Mode
3. Relative strength of contractions; inflection on UA panel of chart paper is made by the contraction of the uterus, which depresses a pressure-sensing button (a thin patient may exhibit large inflections when having only mild contractions; in contrast, an obese patient may exhibit minor inflections when having strong contractions; the nurse must then palpate the abdomen to assess relative strength of contraction)	3. Intensity of contractions (mm Hg pressure at peak of contraction)
	4. Resting tone (mm Hg pressure between contractions)

In a normal labor, uterine contractions occur about every 3 to 5 minutes, with a duration of 30 to 60 seconds, an intensity of 50 to 75 mm Hg, and a resting tone between 5 and 15 mm Hg. In addition to identifying this information, the chart panel also indicates fetal movement by "blips," spikes, or momentary increases in uterine pressure. Identification of fetal movement is important, as it forms the basis for antepartum nonstress testing by identifying fetal reactivity or the presence of accelerations with fetal movement.

During intrapartum monitoring it is important to look for hyperstimulation of the uterus in addition to the frequency, duration, and intensity of contractions and uterine resting tone. Hyperstimulation, as evidenced by increased uterine activity on the chart panel, can result in an asphyxiated fetus (because of interference with the placental circulation) and potentially in uterine rupture. An outlined description of increased uterine activity follows.

Increased Uterine Activity
Observations

1. Contractions lasting longer than 90 seconds
2. Relaxation between contractions less than 30 seconds
3. Inadequate intrauterine relaxation with resting tone above 15 mm Hg between contractions
4. Peak pressure of contractions above 80 mm Hg
5. Contractions more frequent than every 2 minutes

Causes

1. Hyperstimulation of the uterus with oxytocin
2. Abruptio placentae
3. Overdistention of the uterine wall as a result of multiple gestation, hydramnios, or a macrosomic fetus
4. Pregnancy-induced hypertension
5. Drugs
    a. Narcotics (e.g., meperidine hydrochloride [Demerol])
    b. Catecholamines (adrenergics) (e.g., norepinephrine [Noradrenaline, Levarterenol])
    c. Beta-blocking agents (e.g., propranolol [Inderal])
    d. Prostaglandins (e.g., prostaglandin F_2 alpha [$PGF_2\alpha$, Dinoprost])
    e. Pituitary hormones (e.g., vasopressin [Pitressin])
    f. Quinine
    g. Estrogen
    h. Ergonovine
    i. Acetylcholine
    j. Calcium channel blockers

NOTE: A protocol for the induction and augmentation of labor can be found in Appendix B.

Clinical significance

Hyperstimulation of the uterus or a tetanic contraction can result in stress to the fetus, as a result of the lack of placental perfusion and potentially in uterine rupture. The most common cause of uterine hyperstimulation is the injudicious use of oxytocin. When an oxytocin infusion is discontinued, uterine relaxation usually occurs within 10 minutes with return of normal baseline FHR and variability. When oxytocin is given by poorly controlled methods, such as the buccal or intramuscular route, there is an added

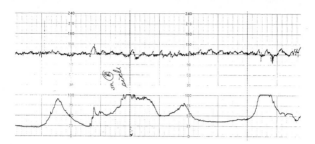

Figure 4-1
Uterine hyperstimulation from oxytocin.

risk because the rate of absorption, as well as any adverse fetal effects, is prolonged (Figure 4-1). A protocol for the administration of oxytocin for induction or augmentation of labor is in Appendix B.

Because uterine contractions are known to decrease the rate of blood flow through the intervillous space and most fetuses are well able to tolerate this transient type of stress, it is important for the nurse to attentively monitor uterine activity, as well as FHR. In pregnancies in which the margin of fetal reserve is low, this phenomenon can cause commensurate decreases in FHR, (described as late decelerations). The physician should be promptly notified when there is evidence of uterine hyperstimulation with or without an associated heart rate response.

Intervention

1. Discontinue oxytocin if infusing (exercise caution in flushing the oxytocin out of the line to ensure that a bolus is not delivered to the patient).
2. Increase rate of maintenance intravenous infusion.
3. Change maternal position (left lateral preferred).
4. Consider administration of oxygen, 8 to 12 L/min by face mask, depending on response in FHR.
5. The physician may consider the use of tocolytics such as terbutaline, magnesium sulfate, or ritodrine if there is an excessive increase in uterine activity, such as tetanic contraction, and a nonreassuring FHR pattern is evident.

Fetal recovery from uterine hypertonus is preferred in utero because once the placental circulation is restored, carbon dioxide from respiratory acidosis, as well as the acidic products of anaerobic metabolism, can be eliminated.

Inhibition of Uterine Activity
Tocolytics

It is important to decrease uterine activity when premature labor or nonreassuring FHR patterns occur. Drugs such as isoxsuprine, epinephrine, and isoproterenol have been used to reduce uterine activity but not without drawbacks (i.e., their beta-stimulant effects cause vasodilation and secondary hypotension). Because of their extrauterine effects, some newer betamimetic agents are now used. Terbutaline and ritodrine are now routinely used because they have maximal uterine relaxant effects and relatively few extrauterine cardiovascular effects, although hypotension can become problematic. In addition magnesium sulfate is frequently considered as the first choice in tocolytic therapy. Other drugs known to inhibit uterine activity include diazoxide, halothane, progesterone, and prostaglandin inhibitors (e.g., ibuprofen).

In the past alcohol had been widely used to successfully stop premature labor in some patients, but in others it has had detrimental results. It is no longer used, however. Alcohol can depress maternal central respiratory and vasomotor centers, inducing secondary hypoxia. It is thought that absolute bed rest alone may be the most valuable treatment in the event of premature labor.

A protocol for the management of preterm labor can be found in Appendix C.

Baseline Fetal Heart Rate

The baseline FHR (Figure 5-1) is that heart rate that occurs when there is no stress or stimulation to the fetus, for example:

1. When the patient is not in labor
2. When the fetus is not moving
3. Between uterine contractions
4. When there is no stimulation to the fetus as occurs with vaginal examinations and electrode application
5. During the interval between periodic changes

The rate is usually between 120 and 160 bpm in the normal full-term fetus. In the premature fetus the heart rate is slightly increased over that occurring at term and the rate is approximately

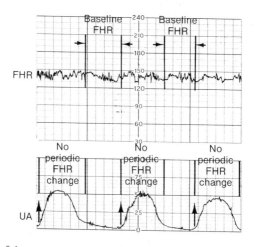

Figure 5-1
Baseline FHR rate is identified between uterine contractions.

160 bpm at about 20 weeks' gestation. The FHR is determined by the atrial pacemaker and balanced in a push-pull relationship by the sympathetic (cardioacceleration) and parasympathetic (cardiodeceleration) divisions of the autonomic nervous system.

Variations in baseline FHR are those that last more than 10 minutes. They are described as tachycardia (increased heart rate), and bradycardia (decreased heart rate). Variability (irregularity in rate from uneven intervals from heartbeat to heartbeat) is the most important FHR characteristic and is a result of the continual push-pull effect of the sympathetic and parasympathetic nervous system.

Tachycardia
Description (Figure 5-2)

Fetal tachycardia is defined as a baseline heart rate above 160 bpm from the normal baseline, which is sustained for a duration of 10 minutes or more. Some individual fetuses may have a normal heart rate in excess of 160 bpm but most likely not more than 170 bpm. Tachycardia should not be confused with acceleration of heart rate, which is a transitory periodic change. When fetal tachycardia occurs, it is generally associated with a decrease in baseline variability, since there is a loss of parasympathetic autonomic activity.

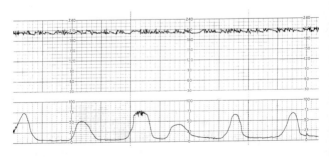

Figure 5-2
Fetal tachycardia.

Causes

1. Early fetal hypoxia	1. Fetus attempts to compensate for reduced blood flow by increase of sympathetic stimulation or release of epinephrine from adrenal medulla, or both
2. Maternal fever	2. Accelerates metabolism of fetal myocardium; increases sympathetic cardioacceleration activity up to 2 hours before the mother is febrile
3. Parasympatholytic drugs (e.g., atropine, scopolamine, hydroxyzine [Vistaril, Atarax], phenothiazines)	3. Block the parasympathetic division of the autonomic nervous system
4. Betasympathomimetic drugs (e.g., ritodrine and isoxsuprine)	4. These tocolytic drugs, given to control labor, have a cardiac stimulant effect similar to that of epinephrine
5. Amnionitis	5. Increased heart rate can be the first sign of developing intrauterine infection (as with prolonged rupture of membranes)
6. Maternal hyperthyroidism	6. Long-acting thyroid stimulating hormones (LATS) probably cross the placenta and increase the fetal heart rate, if maternal hyperthyroidism is controlled
7. Fetal anemia	7. FHR increases in an effort to increase the cardiac output and tissue perfusion
8. Fetal heart failure	8. The fetal heart attempts to compensate for failure by increasing rate and, concurrently, cardiac output; can occur as a result of tachyarrhythmia

9. Fetal cardiac dysrhythmias*

9. Tachyarrhythmias and variations of normal sinus rhythm may occur (e.g., paroxysmal atrial tachycardia [PAT], atrial flutter, and premature ventricular contractions [PVCs]); congenital cardiac anomaly may be present; FHR in excess of 240 bpm cannot be followed by monitor because this exceeds FHR range parameters

Clinical significance

Tachycardia can be an ominous sign when associated with late decelerations, severe variable decelerations, or absence of variability. Persistent tachycardia with average baseline variability or in the absence of periodic changes (e.g., decelerations), does not appear serious in terms of immediate neonatal outcome. This is particularly true when tachycardia is associated with maternal fever.

Sinus tachycardia, atrial flutter/fibrillation, and supraventricular tachycardia are the three types of fetal tachycardia. Sinus tachycardia, with a rate above 160 bpm, is most often caused by a drug effect or is a response to maternal infection such as amnionitis. It is not a sign of fetal hypoxia unless it is associated with late decelerations and/or lack of variability. Atrial flutter/fibrillation with an atrial rate between 300 and 450 bpm is rarely diagnosed in the antepartum period and is associated with a high mortality rate. Supraventricular tachycardia (SVT) with a heart rate in excess of 200 bpm is the most frequently occurring form of fetal tachyarrhythmia. Short periods of SVT are of no clinical significance. However, longer periods of SVT have been associated with high cardiac output failure, nonimmune hydrops fetalis, and fetal death.

Fetal cardiac dysrhythmias may be confused with electrical noise or maternal ECG artifact on the fetal monitor, since they are characterized by large vertical excursions on the FHR scale. They can, however, be diagnosed through the use of abdominal ECG, spiral electrode electrocardiogram, real-time ultrasound, or M-mode ultrasound.

Intervention

Intervention is dependent on etiological factors. Maternal fever can be reduced with antipyretics, hydration, and cooling measures. Oxygen at 8 to 12 L/min may be of some value.

If the diagnosis of SVT is made, such as with M-mode echocardiography, in utero therapy of the immature fetus or delivery of the mature fetus must be initiated. In utero treatment can consist of single drugs or combinations of digoxin, calcium channel blockers (verapamil), beta-blockers (propranolol [Inderal]), and antiarrhythmic agents such as procainamide and quinidine.

Bradycardia
Description (Figure 5-3)

Fetal bradycardia is defined as a baseline heart rate below 120 bpm or less than 30 bpm from the normal baseline for a duration of 10 minutes or more. Some individual fetuses may have a normal heart rate of less than 120 bpm, but most likely not less than 110 bpm. Bradycardia should not be confused with deceleration of heart rate, which is a periodic change. Fetal bradycardia above 90 bpm occurring in the second stage of labor is not considered worrisome unless it is associated with a significant loss of variability.

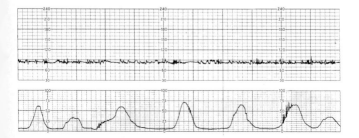

Figure 5-3
Fetal bradycardia.

Causes

1. Late (profound) fetal hypoxia

    1. Myocardial activity becomes depressed and lowers heart rate

2. Beta-adrenergic blocking drugs (e.g., propanolol)

    2. Epinephrine receptor sites in the myocardium are blocked by these drugs, permitting unopposed vagal tone and a decreased heart rate

3. Anesthetics (epidural, spinal, and pudendal)

    3. Bradycardia may develop indirectly because of a reflex mechanism or because of maternal hypotension produced by the drug

4. Maternal hypotension

    4. Maternal supine hypotension syndrome caused by uterine pressure on the vena cava decreases maternal cardiac output and blood pressure and subsequently decreases FHR

5. Prolonged umbilical cord compression

    5. Cord compression activates fetal baroceptors, produces vagal stimulation, and decreases heart rate

6. Fetal cardiac dysrhythmias

    6. FHR can be low (70 to 90 bpm) with bradyarrhythmias (complete heart block)

7. Hypothermia

    7. Maternal (and therefore fetal) hypothermia reduces myocardial metabolism, decreases oxygen requirements, and decreases heart rate

8. Maternal systemic lupus erythematosus

    8. Complete atrioventricular dissociation associated with connective tissue disease produces persistent bradycardia

9. Cytomegalovirus

    9. Bradycardia may be present as a result of congenital heart block from a structural cardiac defect

10. Prolonged maternal hypoglycemia	10. Maternal and subsequently fetal hypoglycemia can potentiate hypoxemia with a depression of myocardial activity and decreased heart rate

Clinical significance

Bradycardia resulting from hypoxia is an ominous sign when associated with loss of variability and late decelerations. Its presence indicates advanced fetal distress and may be a preterminal event. However, bradycardia with average FHR variability and absence of late decelerations is not a sign of fetal distress and should be considered benign. Intervention is also not warranted in fetuses with heart block diagnosed by fetal electrocardiogram in the antepartum period.

Although paracervical blocks are now rarely performed, the resultant bradycardia is usually transitory with recovery occurring in utero. The 5-minute Apgar is usually above 7 if the FHR pattern was reassuring before the onset of bradycardia and if delivery does not occur during the paracervical block bradycardia. Poor fetal outcome has occurred with delivery during bradycardia caused by fetal hypoxia and acidosis. Therefore neonatal resuscitation and stabilization is indicated until the pharmacological agent has been metabolized.

Intervention

Intervention is dependent on etiological factors and clinical judgment based on a variety of factors, including stage of labor and indications of fetal stress. Oxygen at 8 to 12 L/min by face mask may be of some value. Following delivery, a pacemaker may be indicated for some infants with congenital heart block.

Variability
Description

Variability of the FHR can be described as the normal irregularity of cardiac rhythm, resulting from a continuous balancing interaction of the sympathetic (cardioacceleration) and parasympathetic (cardiodeceleration) divisions of the autonomic nervous

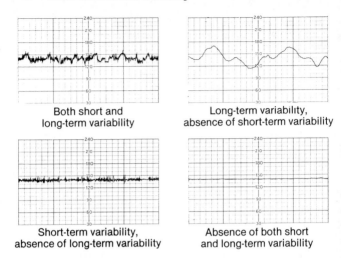

Both short and
long-term variability

Long-term variability,
absence of short-term variability

Short-term variability,
absence of long-term variability

Absence of both short
and long-term variability

Figure 5-4
Variations in short- and long-term variability.

system. These two forces work in a push-pull relationship, modulating the FHR. Good variability on the FHR panel is demonstrated by fluctuations of the FHR baseline. This is indicative of normal neurological control of the heart rate and a measure of fetal reserve.

In contrast, if each interval between heartbeats were exactly the same, as in the regular rhythm of a ticking clock or metronome, the baseline would be flat, indicating central nervous system depression associated with hypoxia. Therefore absence of variability on the FHR panel is demonstrated by a smooth or flat baseline.

Variability is further described as short term or long term. *Short-term variability* is a change in FHR from one beat to the next. This is due to the difference in intervals between consecutive heartbeats. Short-term variability can also be described as the internal difference between successive R peaks of the fetal electrocardiogram (FECG) signal. *Long-term variability* appears as rhythmic fluctuations or waves, generally 3 to 5 cycles per minute and is best assessed over time. Long-term variability is the waviness or cyclic undulations in the baseline rate that is seen over the course of 5 to 10 minutes of a tracing (Figure 5-4 and

Table 5-1). Generally, short- and long-term variability tend to increase and decrease together (Figure 5-5).

Accurate short- and long-term variability are best ensured with the internal mode of monitoring using the spiral electrode.

Table 5-1   Fetal Heart Rate Variability

	Short Term	Long Term
Description	A change in FHR from one beat to the next	Rhythmic and cyclic fluctuations in FHR of 3 to 5 cycles per minute
Appearance		

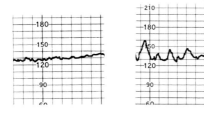

	Short Term	Long Term
Signal source	Spiral electrode; monitors with autocorrelation very closely approximate short-term variability	Internal and external modes of monitoring

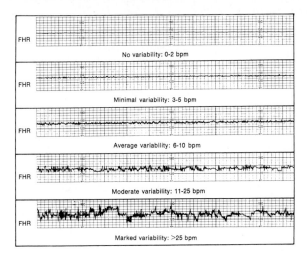

Figure 5-5
FHR variability. Short- and long-term variability tend to increase and decrease together.

External ultrasound most accurately demonstrates long-term variability, but the monitors with autocorrelation very closely approximate short-term variability as evidenced by the simultaneous comparison with monitor strips obtained using the spiral electrode. The external abdominal ECG can assess long-term variability but inconsistently demonstrates short-term variability because of limitations encountered during monitoring, including maternal and fetal coincidental heartbeats, movement, and maternal muscle activity.

Causes of increased variability

1. Early mild hypoxia
2. Fetal stimulation

1. An early compensatory mechanism produces an increase in FHR variability
2. External uterine palpation, uterine contractions, fetal activity, application of spiral electrode, vaginal examination, acoustic stimulation, and maternal activity stimulate the fetal autonomic nervous system resulting in an increase in variability

Causes of decreased variability

1. Hypoxia and acidosis

1. Uteroplacental insufficiency as a result of several causes (uterine hyperstimulation, maternal supine hypotension, pregnancy-induced hypertension, amnionitis). (Other causes are listed under late decelerations, p. 90)

2. Drugs

2. Narcotics, tranquilizers, barbiturates, and anesthetics depress central nervous system mechanisms responsible for cardiac control; anticholinergics such as atropine and scopolamine block the transmission of impulses to the sinoatrial node
Examples follow:
Analgesics/narcotics
Meperidine hydrochloride (Demerol), alphaprodine hydrochloride (Nisentil), morphine sulfate, pentazocine (Talwin)
Barbiturates
Secobarbital sodium (Seconal), pentobarbital sodium (Nembutal), amobarbital (Amytal)
Tranquilizers
Diazepam (Valium)
Phenothiazines
Promethazine hydrochloride (Phenergan), propiomazine hydrochloride (Largon), hydroxyzine pamoate (Vistaril), promazine hydrochloride (Sparine)
Parasympatholytics (Atropine),
General anesthetics

3. Fetal sleep cycles

3. Periods of fetal sleep, usually lasting for 20 to 30 minutes, produce decreased long-term variability; does not usually affect short-term variability

4. Congenital anomalies	4. Central nervous system (e.g., anencephaly) or cardiac anomalies can decrease variability
5. Extreme prematurity	5. Heartbeat is controlled by immature neurological mechanisms, resulting in even intervals from one heart beat to the next
6. Fetal cardiac dysrhythmias	6. Suppression of cardiac control mechanisms may be the result of paroxysmal atrial tachycardia, complete heart block, nodal rhythm, or an aberrant pacemaker

Clinical significance

The significance of marked variability is not known. Increased variability from a previous average variability is thought to be an early sign of mild fetal hypoxia.

Decreasing variability is a warning sign of fetal distress. Absence of variability exhibited by a smooth or flat baseline is a significant sign of fetal distress. It is clearly ominous when associated with late decelerations of *any* magnitude, signifying advanced hypoxia and acidosis related to central nervous system depression. Variability decrease resulting from a drug usually resumes as the drug is excreted. Variability decreased as a result of fetal sleep usually resumes in 20 to 30 minutes.

Variability is considered to be the most important FHR characteristic reflecting appropriate neurological modulation of the FHR. The majority of fetuses with good variability, regardless of deceleration patterns, do well at birth.

Intervention
Increased variability

Observe the FHR tracing carefully for any sign of fetal distress, including decreasing variability and late decelerations. Consider using the internal mode (spiral electrode) of monitoring if the pattern is observed during external monitoring, especially if it is thought to be a precursor of decreased variability.

Decreased variability

Intervention is dependent on the cause. Intervention is not warranted if decreased variability is associated with fetal sleep cycles or if it is temporarily associated with central nervous system depressants. Application of the spiral electrode should be considered if the pattern is observed using external monitoring. If a CNS depressant drug has been given and delivery appears imminent, Narcan may be administered to the mother before delivery and is routinely administered to the neonate after delivery. If hypoxia is suspected, turning the patient on her side and administering oxygen may be of some value.

Summary of Baseline Changes

Tachycardia

Definition	Sustained FHR above 160 bpm or more than 30 bpm above normal baseline for more than 10 minutes
Etiology	Early fetal hypoxia, drugs, maternal fever, amnionitis, fetal anemia, fetal heart failure, and/or cardiac arrhythmias
Clinical significance	Usually benign when associated with maternal fever
	Nonreassuring when associated with late decelerations, loss of variability, or severe variable decelerations
Nursing intervention	Dependent on etiological factors; lateral position change and oxygen at 8 to 12 L/min may be of some value; reduce maternal fever with hydration antipyretics and cooling measures

Bradycardia	Minimal to Absent Variability
Sustained FHR below 120 bpm or more than 30 bpm below normal baseline for more than 10 minutes	*Short term*: changes in FHR from one beat to the next *Long term:* rhythmic fluctuations in the baseline about 3 to 5 cycles per minute
Late (profound) fetal hypoxia, drugs, maternal hypotension, prolapsed cord, or congenital heart block	*Decreased variability:* prematurity, drugs, hypoxia, fetal sleep, congenital abnormalities, fetal cardiac arrhythmias, CNS depression
Bradycardia without periodic deceleration and with average FHR variability is not a sign of fetal hypoxia	Benign when associated with periodic fetal sleep; return of variability usually occurs when drugs are excreted or metabolized
Ominous when associated with late decelerations or loss of variability; indicates profound fetal distress	Ominous when associated with late decelerations
Dependent on etiological factors; lateral position change and oxygen at 8 to 12 L/min may be of some value; intervention is not warranted in fetus with heart block diagnosed by ECG in the antepartum period	Dependent on etiological factors; fetal blood sampling for pH may provide additional clinical information; intervention is not warranted if associated with fetal sleep cycle or temporarily associated with central nervous system depressants

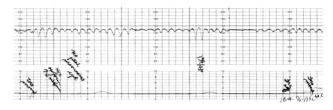

Figure 5-6
Sinusoidal FHR.
(Courtesy Roger K. Freeman, M.D., Long Beach, Calif.)

Unusual Patterns
Sinusoidal pattern (Figure 5-6)

A sinusoidal fetal heart rate pattern is characterized by the following features:

1. A heart rate between 120 and 160 bpm
2. Regular oscillations with an amplitude of 5 to 15 bpm
3. Frequency of 2 to 5 cycles per minute of long-term variability
4. Minimal to absent short-term variability
5. Rhythmic oscillation of a sine wave above and below a baseline
6. Absence of FHR accelerations in response to fetal movement

This pattern has been known to occur in the presence of fetal hypoxia, often as a result of Rh isoimmunization, fetal anemia, and chronic fetal bleeds. In these cases it has been associated with an increase in fetal morbidity and mortality, and survival may depend on extrauterine support in a neonatal intensive care unit.

The pattern has also been reported after the administration of analgesics, such as alphaprodine (Nisentil), meperidine (Demerol), and butorphanol tartrate (Stadol), and in association with amnionitis. The sinusoidal pattern following the administration of these drugs is usually a temporary phenomenon and is not associated with an adverse fetal outcome.

Expeditious delivery may be indicated if there is a persistent, uncorrectable sinusoidal pattern and other signs of fetal distress are present. If the pattern is inconsistent and apparently transitory after intravenous narcotics, fetal compromise is not expected.

Lambda pattern

A lambda pattern is one in which an acceleration is followed immediately by a deceleration. This pattern is fairly common, not associated with fetal distress, but important to distinguish from late decelerations or other abnormal patterns. It often appears early in labor and does not persist throughout the entire labor period.

Fetal cardiac dysrhythmias

Fetal cardiac dysrhythmias occur in many pregnancies and fall into the following descriptive categories:

1. Fetal tachycardia

   1. Sinus tachycardia, atrial flutter/fibrillation, and supraventricular tachycardia are described on p. 68.

2. Fetal bradycardia

   2. Congenital heart block of first, second, or third degree can result in bradycardia. First-degree block does not require treatment in the fetus and has not yet been reported in the literature. In second-degree block not all the impulses from the sinoatrial node in the atria are conducted to the ventricles. Mobitz type I block is evidenced by a progressive lengthening of the PR interval and is rarely of any significance. Mobitz type II block occurs infrequently but is more serious and often a precursor to third-degree heart block. This is described in the section on fetal bradycardia on p. 71.

3. Premature atrial contractions (PACs) and premature significance ventricular contractions (PVCs)

   3. These are represented on the tracing as vertical excursions above or below the FHR baseline. PACs and PVCs usually have no clinical significance and do not require intervention.

4. Transient fetal cardiac asystole

4. Transient fetal cardiac arrest may be evidenced by a rapid downward deflection of the FHR followed quickly by a rapid upward excursion back to the previous FHR baseline. This has been reported during the nadir of severe variable decelerations. Management should include position change, vaginal examination to rule out cord prolapse or rapid fetal descent, and elevation of the presenting part as indicated.

It is important to distinguish fetal dysrhythmias from electrical noise or maternal ECG artifact, since they can all be evidenced by the same pattern. To adequately discriminate fetal dysrhythmias from noise and artifact, diagnoses can be achieved by abdominal ECG, spiral electrode electrocardiogram, real-time ultrasound, and M-mode ultrasound.

Periodic Changes

Periodic changes in FHR are transient accelerations or decelerations from the baseline, with the FHR returning to the baseline. They usually occur in response to uterine contractions but can also occur with stimulation such as fetal movement. They are classified as accelerations and early, late, and variable decelerations.

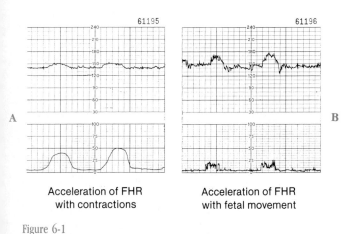

Acceleration of FHR
with contractions

Acceleration of FHR
with fetal movement

Figure 6-1
A, Acceleration of FHR with uterine contractions. **B,** Acceleration of FHR with fetal movement.

Accelerations
Description

Accelerations of FHR from the baseline, are most often associated with fetal movement and uterine contractions. They can also occur before or after variable decelerations. Accelerations are transitory increases above the baseline and may resemble the shape of uterine contractions. The onset is variable, often preceding or occurring simultaneously with uterine contractions or fetal movement. The recovery is variable and the amplitude is usually 15 or more bpm from the baseline (Figure 6-1).

Characteristics

	Spontaneous	Uniform
SHAPE	Does not necessarily resemble shape of uterine contraction	Resembles shape of uterine contraction
ONSET	Variable, can occur anytime	Before or after peak of uterine contraction
RECOVERY	Variable	Return to baseline can occur after or at the same time as the uterine pressure returns to its resting tone
ACCELERATION	Usually above 15 bpm	Variable; usually 10 to 15 bpm
BASELINE	Usually associated with average baseline variability	Sometimes associated with decreasing or smooth baseline variability
OCCURRENCE	Variable; not associated with uterine contraction or periodic decelerations; in response to fetal stimulation	Repetitious; tends to occur with each contraction; has occurred in some cases before the onset of late decelerations

Etiology

Stimulation of the sympathetic division of the autonomic nervous system can accelerate the FHR. Acceleration can result from the following:

1. Spontaneous fetal movement
2. Vaginal examination
3. Electrode application
4. Breech presentation
5. Occiput posterior presentation
6. Uterine contractions
7. Fundal pressure
8. Abdominal palpation

Clinical significance

Spontaneous acceleration of FHR of ≥ 15 bpm for ≥ 15 seconds in response to fetal movement and uterine contractions is an indication of fetal central nervous system (CNS) alertness and well-being and is reassuring. Fetal movement can be observed on the uterine activity panel as spikes or momentary increases in uterine pressure on the lower section of the monitor strip.

Uniform accelerations occurring with uterine contractions on a repetitive basis may be the earliest indicator of possible partial cord compression.

Intervention

Acceleration of FHR is considered a benign pattern, and no intervention is required. However, it would be wise to observe uniform accelerations just in case they are followed by a small deceleration that can evolve into a pattern of variable or late decelerations as labor progresses.

Early Decelerations
Description

Early decelerations are those that begin early in the contracting phase with the onset before the peak of the uterine contraction and the recovery occurring at the same time the uterine contraction returns to the baseline. The timing is synchronous with that of the contraction.

Physiology

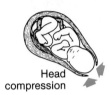

Head compression

Pressure on the fetal skull
↓
Alters cerebral blood flow
↓
Stimulates central vagus nerve
↓
Produces decrease in heart rate with
↓
Recovery occurring as pressure is re-lieved

Characteristics (Figure 6-2)

SHAPE	Uniform shape; a "mirror image" of the contraction phase
ONSET	Early in the contraction phase; before the peak of the contraction; nadir, or low point, of the deceleration occurs at the peak of the contraction
RECOVERY	Return to baseline occurs by the end of the contraction as uterine pressure returns to its resting tone
DECELERATION	Rarely decelerates below 100 bpm, or 20 to 30 bpm below baseline; amplitude of deceleration is usually proportional to amplitude of contraction
BASELINE	Usually associated with average baseline variability
OCCURRENCE	Repetitious; occurs with each contraction; usually observed between 4 and 7 cm dilatation and, in second stage, as fetal head descends through pelvis

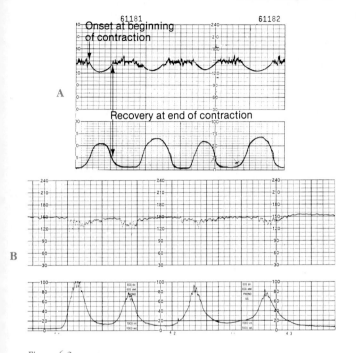

Figure 6-2
A, Early deceleration (illustration with key points identified). **B,** Early deceleration (actual tracing).

Etiology

Head compression can result from the following:
1. Uterine contractions
2. Vaginal examination
3. Fundal pressure
4. Placement of the internal mode of fetal monitoring

Clinical significance

Early deceleration has no pathological significance. It is a benign pattern not associated with fetal hypoxia or acidosis. It is not usually associated with tachycardia or other heart rate changes.

Intervention

Early deceleration is a benign pattern and no intervention is required. The importance of identifying early decelerations is to be able to distinguish them from late and variable decelerations.

Late Decelerations
Description

Late decelerations are those that begin late in the contracting phase with the onset at or after the peak of the uterine contraction and the recovery occurring after the return of the contraction to the baseline. They are generally proportional to uterine contractions and thus are readily observed with stronger contractions and not as evident with weaker contractions.

Physiology

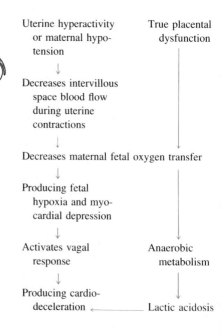

Uteroplacental insufficiency

Uterine hyperactivity or maternal hypotension
↓
Decreases intervillous space blood flow during uterine contractions
↓
Decreases maternal fetal oxygen transfer
↓
Producing fetal hypoxia and myocardial depression
↓
Activates vagal response
↓
Producing cardiodeceleration ←——————

True placental dysfunction

Anaerobic metabolism
↓
Lactic acidosis

Characteristics (Figure 6-3)

SHAPE	Uniform shape; a "mirror image" of the contraction phase
ONSET	Late in the contraction phase at or after the peak of the contraction; nadir, or low point, of the deceleration occurs well after the peak of the contraction
RECOVERY	Return to the baseline occurs after the end of the contraction (usually more than 20 seconds after uterine pressure returns to its resting tone)
DECELERATION	Rarely decelerates below 100 bpm; amplitude of deceleration is usually proportional to amplitude of contraction; *persistent, uncorrected* decelerations of *any* magnitude are ominous, and the most depressed fetuses may have only shallow late decelerations (e.g., 3 to 5 bpm)
BASELINE	Often associated with loss of variability and a rising baseline or tachycardia; variability may be increased during the nadir of the deceleration
OCCURRENCE	Repetitious; occurs with each contraction; can be observed at any time during labor when there is uteroplacental insufficiency

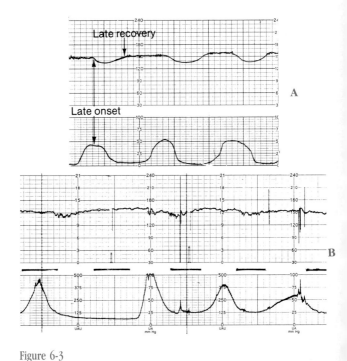

Figure 6-3
A, Late deceleration (illustration with key points identified).
B, Late decelerations (actual tracing).

Etiology

Uteroplacental insufficiency can result from the following:

1. Hyperstimulation of the uterus from oxytocin augmentation or induction

2. Maternal supine hypotension

3. Pregnancy-induced hypertension

4. Chronic hypertension

5. Postmaturity

6. Amnionitis

1. Hyperstimulation enhances vasoconstriction, reduces cardiac output, and decreases intervillous space blood flow

2. Compression of the inferior vena cava reduces venous return and maternal cardiac output

3. Vasospasm occurring in uterine vessels decreases intervillous space blood flow and produces fetal hypoxia

4. Hypertensive vascular disease constricts blood vessels and reduces intervillous blood flow, thus producing fetal hypoxia

5. Fetus "outgrows" placenta; insufficient function of the placenta reduces supply of oxygen and nutrients to the fetus

6. Maternal infection reduces the efficiency of the uteroplacental unit; related fetal tachycardia increases the metabolic rate, rapidly depleting placental oxygen reserves; amnionitis often causes uterine hyperactivity, which decreases intervillous space blood flow and leads to fetal hypoxia

7. Small-for-gestational-age (SGA)	7. Intrauterine growth retardation (IUGR) with reduced fetal placental reserve
8. Maternal diabetes	8. Maternal vascular involvement and sclerotic arterial changes reduce uteroplacental perfusion
9. Placenta previa	9. Placental attachment to the lower uterine segment (covering internal cervical os) may cause early separation and increase chance of hemorrhage
10. Abruptio placentae	10. Premature separation of placenta decreases functioning placental area and related uterine hyperactivity
11. Conduction anesthetics (spinal, caudal, epidural, and saddle)	11. May cause maternal hypotension, reducing blood flow to uteroplacental unit
12. Maternal cardiac disease	12. Conditions that affect pumping of blood reduce blood flow to uteroplacental unit; cyanotic conditions reduce oxygen content of blood flowing to placenta
13. Maternal anemia	13. Reduction of RBCs or hemoglobin decreases the amount of oxygen to fetoplacental unit
14. Rh isoimmunization	14. Fetal anemia decreases the amount of available oxygen and the hypoxic stress occurring with U.C. can precipitate metabolic acidosis
15. Other conditions; collagen vascular disease, renal disease and advanced maternal age	15. Conditions compromise placental exchange because of sclerotic arterial and venous changes

Clinical significance

Late decelerations of any magnitude should be considered a worrisome sign when they are persistent and uncorrectable. When
they are associated with tachycardia and/or minimal or absent
variability they can be an ominous sign. As myocardial depression increases, the depth of the late deceleration decreases, becoming more subtle or shallow in appearance. In contrast, a single late deceleration in an otherwise reassuring pattern is not
clinically significant.

Persistent and uncorrectable late decelerations reflect repetitive hypoxic stress and if associated with minimal or absent variability become a sign of increasing metabolic acidosis.

Intervention

Procedure*	Rationale
1. Change maternal position (left lateral is preferred)	1. Decreases pressure on the inferior vena cava and corrects supine hypotension
2. Correct maternal hypotension	2.
a. Elevate legs (particularly after conduction anesthetics)	a. Increases venous return and promotes cardiac output
b. Increase rate of maintenance IV infusion	b. Increases maternal circulating volume and cardiac output; this can facilitate excretion of oxytocin
3. Discontinue oxytocin if infusing	3. Decreases uterine activity
4. Administer oxygen 8 to 12 L/min by face mask	4. Increases maternal oxygen saturation of hemoglobin
5. Fetal scalp or acoustic stimulation	5. May be useful to elicit an acceleration of FHR that would not be indicative of fetal acidosis

*Consider placement of internal electrode as appropriate for better assessment of
potential problems.

6. Termination of labor is considered by the physician if the pattern cannot be corrected, particularly if variability is decreasing and an acceleration of FHR cannot be elicited

6. Continuation of labor can only further compromise the fetus by increasing hypoxia and acidosis

Variable Decelerations
Description

Variable decelerations are those occurring anytime during the uterine contracting phase but are often concurrent with uterine contractions. The decelerations vary in intensity and duration and frequently decelerate below the average FHR range. Variable deceleration patterns are the most frequently observed FHR pattern in labor.

Physiology

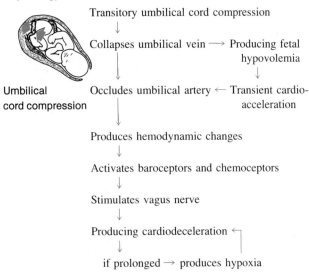

Transitory umbilical cord compression
↓
Collapses umbilical vein ⟶ Producing fetal hypovolemia
↓   ↓
Umbilical cord compression   Occludes umbilical artery ← Transient cardio-acceleration
↓
Produces hemodynamic changes
↓
Activates baroceptors and chemoceptors
↓
Stimulates vagus nerve
↓
Producing cardiodeceleration ←┐
↓   │
if prolonged ⟶ produces hypoxia

Characteristics

SHAPE

Variable; does not reflect the shape of any associated uterine contraction; characterized by a sudden drop in heart rate in a ⎺\/⎺ or ⎽_/⎺ shape

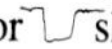

ONSET

Variable times in the contraction phase; often preceded by transitory acceleration (shouldering)

RECOVERY

Return to baseline occurs rapidly, sometimes with transitory acceleration (shouldering), \/\/ or ⎯\/ "overshoot"

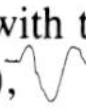

DECELERLATION

Often decelerates below 100 bpm

BASELINE

May be associated with average baseline variability

OCCURRENCE

Not necessarily repetitive; frequently observed late in labor; may be associated with pushing in the second stage of labor

Variations (Figures 6-4 to 6-6)

Mild: decelerates to any level less than 30 seconds with abrupt return to baseline

Moderate: decelerates no less than 80 bpm, any duration with abrupt return to baseline

Severe: decelerates below 70 bpm for greater than 45 to 60 seconds with slow return to baseline (baseline rate may increase while baseline variability decreases)

Etiology

Umbilical cord compression can result from the following:

1. Maternal position; cord between fetus and maternal pelvis
2. Cord around fetal neck, leg, arm, or other body part
3. Short cord
4. Knot in cord
5. Prolapsed cord

Clinical Significance

Variable decelerations occur in about 50% of all labors and are usually transient and correctable phenomena.

Reassuring variable decelerations:

1. Last no more than 30 to 45 seconds
2. Have a rapid return to baseline from the nadir of the deceleration
3. Retain normal short-term variability and normal baseline rate continues

Transitory umbilical cord compression is associated with respiratory acidosis, which is rapidly corrected when cord compression is relieved.

Shouldering or a transitory acceleration of the FHR preceding and following the deceleration indicates a minor degree of cord compression and interaction of the sympathetic and parasympa-

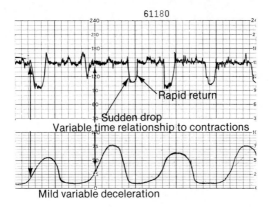

Figure 6-4
Mild variable decelerations (illustration with key points identified).

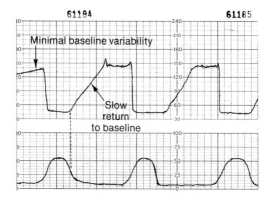

Figure 6-5
Severe variable decelerations (illustration with key points identified).

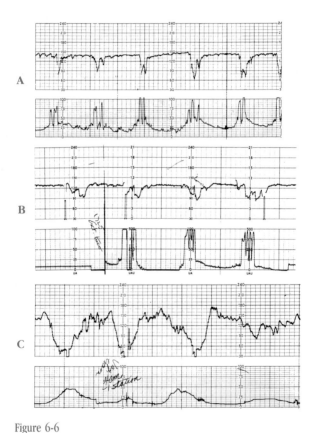

Figure 6-6

A, Mild variable deceleration. **B,** Moderate variable
deceleration. **C,** Severe variable decelerations (all are actual
tracings).

thetic divisions of the autonomic nervous system. Shouldering is generally associated with normal or increased variability.

Severe variable decelerations just before delivery are usually well tolerated if the total time is short from the onset of the decelerations to the time of delivery, and if the neonate is able to eliminate excess respiratory carbon dioxide.

An "overshoot" or smooth transitory acceleration of the FHR upon return of decelerated FHR to baseline indicates that a significant hypoxic stress has occurred. Overshoots generally follow variable decelerations with absent variability.

A progressively slower return to baseline with repetitive variable decelerations indicates a gradual increase in hypoxia. Severe uncorrectable variable decelerations, particularly with loss of short-term variability and a rise in baseline rate, are associated with fetal acidosis, hypoxia, and a neurologically depressed newborn.

Intervention

Procedure*	Rationale
1. Additional intervention for mild variable decelerations is not necessary	1. Pattern is reassuring and does not pose a threat to fetus
2. Change maternal position from side to side, Trendelenburg, or knee-chest	2. May relieve cord compression
3. When decelerations are severe:	3. Pattern may be a warning or ominous sign of fetal distress
a. Discontinue oxytocin if infusing	a. Decreases uterine activity, which can contribute to cord compression
b. Administer oxygen 8 to 12 L/min by face mask	b. Increases maternal oxygen saturation of hemoglobin in an attempt to raise fetal Po_2 when cord is decompressed

*Consider placement of internal electrode as appropriate for better assessment of potential problems.

Procedure	Rationale
c. Vaginal or speculum examination, or both	c. Checks for prolapsed umbilical cord or imminent delivery
d. Amnioinfusion may be of some value	d. Instillation of normal saline through the intrauterine catheter may relieve cord compression (See Chapter 7)
e. Termination of labor is considered by the physician if the severe variable deceleration pattern cannot be corrected. (If the pattern is corrected enough to be reassuring, the labor can be allowed to continue)	e. Continuation of severe variable decelerations can only further compromise the fetus by increasing hypoxia and acidosis

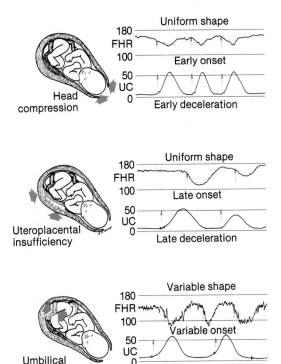

Figure 6-7
Summary of periodic changes.

Summary of Periodic Changes: Decelerations (Figure 6-7)

	Early
Etiology	Head compression
Onset	Early; before peak of uterine contraction (UC)
Recovery	By end of contraction as uterine pressure returns to resting tone
Deceleration	Rarely decelerates below 100 bpm
Clinical significance	Benign
Nursing intervention	None

Late	Variable
Uteroplacental insufficiency	Cord compression
Late; at or after peak of UC, with nadir, or low point, well after peak of UC	Variable; anytime between or during contractions
After end of UC, well after pressure has returned to resting tone	Variable; may have rapid return, prolonged return, "overshoot," or shouldering over baseline
Can decelerate any amount but is usually within normal FHR range of 120 to 160 bpm	Often decelerates below normal FHR range
Ominous	Usually transient but can be ominous
Change maternal position	Change maternal position
Correct maternal hypotension; elevate legs; increase rate of maintenance IV infusion	Continue with the following only for severe variable decelerations:
Discontinue oxytocin if infusing	Discontinue oxytocin if infusing
Administer oxygen 8 to 12 L/min by face mask	Administer oxygen 8 to 12 L/min by face mask
Fetal scalp or acoustic stimulation, pH, or termination of labor may be indicated	Vaginal or speculum examination, or both; amnioinfusion; termination of labor may be indicated if severe variable decelerations are not correctable

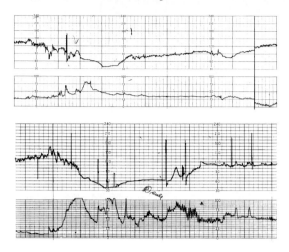

Figure 6-8
Prolonged declerations.

Prolonged Decelerations
Description

Generally a prolonged deceleration is an isolated event. It is most frequently associated with occult or frank cord prolapse and progressive severe variable decelerations. It is characterized by a prolonged deceleration of 60 to 90 seconds or more below the average FHR range.

Characteristics (Figure 6-8)

SHAPE	Variable in shape; does not reflect the shape of any associated uterine contraction
ONSET	Variable times in the contracting phase
RECOVERY	May last 90 seconds or more, with a loss of variability and rebound tachycardia; occasionally a period of late decelerations follows; some fetuses do not recover and the result is fetal death

DECELERATION	Deceleration is almost always below the normal FHR range
BASELINE	Often associated with a loss of variability and postdeceleration tachycardia
OCCURRENCE	Usually isolated events but may be seen late in the course of repetitive, severe variable decelerations or during a prolonged series of late decelerations and just before fetal death

Etiology

1. Cord compression

1. A sudden occult or frank prolapse of umbilical cord

2. Maternal hypotension (supine or related to epidural or spinal anesthesia)

2. Profound uteroplacental insufficiency may result from hypotension, causing a prolonged deceleration

3. Paracervical anesthesia

3. Possibly related to fetal uptake of anesthetic agent, local hypotension from uterine artery spasms, or uterine hypertonus

4. Tetanic uterine contractions (oxytocin stimulation, abruptio placentae, or related to epidural anesthesia)

4. Hypertonic contractions result in uteroplacental insufficiency; inadvertent intravenous injection of anesthetic with an epidural block can result in a tetanic contraction and prolonged deceleration; breast hyperstimulation; *cocaine ingestion* with vasospasm, hypertonus, and abruptio placentae

5. Maternal hypoxia

5. Maternal seizure activity or respiratory depression (from narcotic overdose, magnesium sulfate, or high spinal anesthetic)

6. Procedures and physiological mechanisms: spiral electrode application; pelvic examination; sustained maternal Valsalva; rapid fetal descent through the birth canal

6. Fetal head compression/ stimulation can produce a strong vagal response, cardiodeceleration, and a prolonged deceleration

Clinical significance

Prolonged deceleration(s) associated with fetal head compression (spiral electrode application, pelvic examination, sustained maternal Valsalva, rapid fetal descent) usually lasts for only 1 to 2 minutes and recovers with predeceleration variability and baseline. Decelerations caused by maternal hypotension, tetanic contractions, and maternal hypoxia generally recover with some loss of variability, and tachycardia or recurrent late decelerations. If a subsequent prolonged deceleration does not recur, the placenta generally recovers the fetus to its predeceleration state. The prognosis for fetal survival is guarded if the prolonged deceleration occurs after a series of repetitive severe variable decelerations. In this situation prolonged deceleration and/or recurrent late decelerations may result in a terminal bradycardia of 30 to 60 bpm before death.

 Intervention

Intervention is entirely based on alleviating the cause, which may include "waiting it out" to ensure that fetal recovery occurs. However, if the apparent cause is severe uteroplacental insufficiency, umbilical cord compression, or is unidentifiable, then expeditious delivery may be indicated. Measures used to treat fetal distress can be instituted in any case, and these are described in detail under the topic "Intervention for Fetal Distress" in Chapter 7.

Fetal Distress

7

The focus of electronic FHR monitoring is to identify the earliest stages of fetal hypoxia and appropriately intervene to prevent fetal asphyxia, which can result from sustained and severe hypoxia. To do this, a knowledge of reassuring, suspicious, and nonreassuring patterns is essential to appropriate interventions. Before reviewing these patterns it must be stated that there is no generally agreed upon precise definition of fetal distress. Hypoxia is considered to be a reduction of oxygen supply to tissue below physiological levels, while asphyxia is the end result of profound hypoxia, resulting in anaerobic metabolism and resultant metabolic acidosis.

The diagnosis of birth asphyxia on the basis of fetal pH, Apgar score, and newborn cerebral dysfunction has been described by Gilstrap et al. and should only be applied in the clinical condition defined by the following:

1. Profound umbilical artery metabolic or mixed acidemia (pH < 7.00, base deficit > 20)
2. Five-minute Apgar score of 0 to 3
3. Neonatal neurological sequelae such as seizures, coma, and hypotonia
4. Multiorgan system dysfunction such as the cardiovascular, gastrointestinal, hematologic, renal, and/or pulmonary systems

Although electronic fetal monitoring was intended to be used as a reflector of the adequacy of fetal oxygenation and not to reflect brain function, there are some fetal heart rate patterns that have been described as usually consistent with existing fetal brain damage. These include the following:

1. A flat tracing without late decelerations, variable decelerations, or prolonged bradycardia has been described with anencephaly (vanderMoer et al., Dicker et al., and deHaan et al.).

2. A wandering pattern of blunt, slow, irregular undulations with a flat baseline has been reported with anencephaly (Freeman and Garite).

3. A sinusoidal EFM pattern has been described in cases of hydrocephalus (Ombelet and VanDer Merwe).

4. A fixed heart rate or one with late decelerations, or both, and terminal bradycardias have been reported to occur in fetuses with severe CNS anomalies. (Didolkar and Mutch).

5. A (a) fixed heart rate of 150 bpm with no accelerations or decelerations and a (b) normal tracing except for a 20-minute interval of late decelerations were reported in two infants with typical neonatal hypoxic ischemic encephalopathy but with completely normal umbilical artery blood gas levels (Menticoglou et al.).

6. A normal baseline rate with absent variability and mild variable decelerations with overshoot have been reported in fetuses with preexisting fetal brain damage (Shields and Schifrin).

In addition to the foregoing, there is a consensus that an abnormal EFM tracing is a poor predictor of cerebral palsy (CP), even though EFM can identify fetal asphyxia, which can subsequently result in CP. Although this may seem contradictory, in reality (1) EFM can fail to detect severe fetal asphyxia in an undetermined number of cases, (2) perinatal asphyxia is an uncommon cause of CP (possible causes include congenital developmental defects, intrauterine infection, intrauterine exposure to toxins and teratogens, hypothyroidism, and neonatal asphyxia [Hankins]), and (3) EFM changes that reflect fetal asphyxia and/or acidosis may be the result of a damaged fetal brain and may be a consequence instead of the cause of CP (Niswander).

In conclusion, the focus of electronic FHR monitoring is to identify patterns that are reassuring and predictive of a positive fetal outcome. To do this, a knowledge of reassuring, suspicious, and nonreassuring patterns is essential to prompt and appropriate interventions. This chapter describes patterns associated with fetal distress after describing those patterns that are reassuring and considered normal.

Normal (Reassuring) Fetal Heart Rate Patterns

A reassuring fetal heart rate pattern is one that is in the average FHR range of 120 to 160 bpm without tachycardia or bradycardia, demonstrates average short- and long-term variability when electronically monitored, is reactive in that there are FHR accelerations with fetal movement, and electronically displays an absence of periodic late and nonreassuring variable decelerations.

Description

Baseline Rate	120 to 160 bpm
Short-term variability	More than 6 bpm in amplitude
Long-term variability	3 to 5 cycles per minute
Periodic changes	Accelerations with fetal movement; early decelerations; reassuring variable decelerations
(Figure 7-1)	

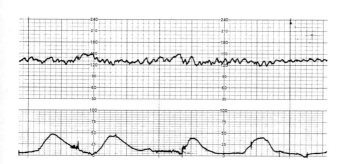

Figure 7-1
Normal FHR and uterine activity pattern.

Normal Uterine Activity Pattern

Frequency	More than 2 minutes between contractions
Duration	Less than 90 seconds
Intensity	Less than 100 mm Hg pressure
Resting tone	Thirty seconds or more between contractions; resting intrauterine pressure less than 15 mm Hg (can be determined only by intrauterine monitoring)

A reassuring FHR and uterine activity pattern serves to allay the concerns of the patient and staff about the fetal status. This type of pattern indicates that the fetus is tolerating the process of labor well and does not require any type of intervention. One would expect to have a good fetal outcome with normal Apgar scores and blood gases.

Suspicious Fetal Heart Rate Patterns

Suspicious or warning fetal heart rate patterns may be self-limiting, or they may be forerunners of nonreassuring FHR patterns. Therefore they should be observed preferably by the direct method of monitoring with a spiral electrode until the pattern becomes reassuring or until intervention for a nonreassuring pattern is indicated. Suspicious patterns include the following:

- Progressive increase or decrease in baseline FHR
- Tachycardia of 160 bpm or more than 30 bpm from previous baseline
- Decreasing baseline variability without any known cause

Nonreassuring Fetal Heart Rate Patterns and Interventions (Figure 7-2)

Intervention for nonreassuring or worrisome FHR patterns should be done in a step-by-step approach, and one should proceed to the next step only if the pattern is uncorrected.

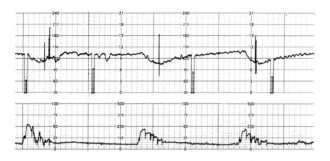

Figure 7-2
Nonreassuring FHR pattern.

Nonreassuring Fetal Heart Rate Patterns	Intervention
Severe variable deceleration: FHR below 70 bpm, lasting longer than 30 to 45 seconds with any of the following: Rising baseline FHR Decreasing variability Slow return to baseline; may be with "overshoot"	With severe variable deceleration: Change maternal position
	Perform vaginal or speculum examination, or both
	Discontinue oxytocin if infusing (consider tocolysis)
	Administer oxygen at 8 to 12 L/min by face mask
	Amnioinfusion may be considered
	Termination of labor should be considered if pattern cannot be corrected enough to meet criteria of mild deceleration
Late decelerations of any magnitude, more serious if associated with decreasing variability or rising baseline	Intervene in step-by-step approach, proceeding to next step *only* if pattern is uncorrected
	Place patient on side (left lateral is preferred)
	Elevate patient's legs
	Increase rate of maintenance IV infusion

Purpose	Rationale
To relieve pressure on the umbilical cord	Improves umbilical blood flow
To rule out a prolapsed cord	Continue other interventions or set up for a cesarean delivery if cord is prolapsed
To reduce repetitive pressure on cord	Discontinue exogenous source of uterine stimulation
To promote maternal hyperoxia	Increases available oxygen to the fetus
To relieve pressure on the umbilical cord	Correct oligohydramnios
To correct supine hypotension	Remove the weight of the fetus from the inferior vena cava, which then allows better blood return to the heart, increasing maternal cardiac output and subsequently blood pressure
To correct maternal hypotension	Diminishes pooling of blood in extremities and increase circulating volume
To correct maternal hypotension	Increases circulating blood volume

Nonreassuring Fetal Heart Rate Patterns	Intervention
	Discontinue oxytocin if infusing (consider tocolysis) (do this first if uterine hyperstimulation is present)
	Administer oxygen at 8 to 12 L/min by face mask
	Stimulate fetal scalp or give sound stimulation
Absence of variability	Correct identifiable cause
Prolonged deceleration	As above
Severe bradycardia	As above

Purpose	Rationale
To reduce uterine activity	Decreases strength and frequency of uterine contractions, which can improve uteroplacental blood flow
To promote maternal hyperoxia	Increases fetal oxygenation
To identify FHR reactivity (increase of FHR 15 bpm in response to stimulus)	Indicates fetal well-being Expeditious delivery should be considered if pattern cannot be corrected

Other Methods of Assessment
Meconium

The presence or absence of meconium is now known not to be a reliable indicator of fetal condition, even though it has been used as such for many centuries. It is estimated that 12% of all fetuses pass meconium before delivery. There are many fetuses with meconium in the amniotic fluid that do not show signs of hypoxia; however, term neonates who are asphyxiated at birth have usually passed meconium. The passage of meconium late in labor in association with fetal heart rate abnormalities has been shown to be a warning sign of possible fetal distress; therefore the FHR pattern needs to be continually assessed and appropriate interventions performed.

To ensure that meconium is not aspirated by the neonate, special care should be taken during the delivery process. The nasopharynx and oropharynx should be suctioned immediately as the head is being delivered. The mother may need to be instructed to blow repetitively to refrain from pushing to allow for suctioning to occur before the neonate takes its first breath. Following delivery the neonate should be subject to endotracheal intubation and tracheal suctioning until the meconium is cleared. All of these procedures should be clearly described in the patient's record by the person performing them.

Fetal heart rate response to stimulation

Stimulation of the fetus to elicit an acceleration of FHR for at least 15 seconds has been reported as an alternative to scalp pH testing, a discussion of which is found in the next section. Several studies have correlated the fetal scalp pH with the FHR response to a stimulus and have attested to the efficacy of these mechanisms. These include the following:

1. *Scalp stimulation:* Digital pressure of the scalp for a 15-second period, followed by application of an atraumatic Allis clamp to the scalp for 15 seconds
2. *Sound stimulation:* Vibroacoustic stimulation by placing an artificial larynx on the maternal abdomen over the fetal head (described fully on p. 128)

The rationale for these mechanisms is that if an acceleration of 15 bpm for 15 seconds occurs with the stimulation, one can assume that the fetal pH is normal. Studies have shown that no less than 50% of stimulated fetuses will have an FHR acceleration, and this is highly predictive of fetal well-being and a pH of no less than 7.25. Of the fetuses that do not accelerate, about one half are not acidotic; therefore absence of an acceleration to the stimulus is not totally predictive of an abnormal pH, fetal acidosis, or fetal distress.

Fetal Blood Sampling for Acid-Base Monitoring

Fetal blood sampling was first described by Saling in 1962 as a means of identifying fetal hypoxemia and acidosis. A decrease in blood pH becomes a measure of the degree of hypoxia, as a result of a change occurring from aerobic to anaerobic metabolism when the fetus is faced with hypoxia. This results in the production of lactic acid and a subsequent drop in pH.

A small amount of fetal blood is obtained from the skin of the presenting part—usually the fetal scalp. To measure P_{O_2}, P_{CO_2}, and base deficit, a larger sample of fetal blood is required. Because these values do not provide enough additional information to warrant their measurement, and because blood gas values can vary so rapidly with transient circulatory changes, the use of fetal blood sampling during the intrapartum period is not routinely warranted. Various factors can influence pH during the intrapartum-predelivery period, and make values disproportionate to the condition at birth. These factors are listed as follows:

1. Maternal acidosis or alkalosis
2. Laboratory errors in determination
3. Caput succedaneum ($\downarrow$ pH value)
4. Stage of labor
5. Time relationship of scalp sampling to uterine contractions
6. Influence of in utero treatment
7. Transience of the insult causing fetal acidosis (metabolic acidosis is less readily reversible than respiratory acidosis)
8. Contamination of sample with amniotic fluid ($\downarrow$ pH value) or room air ($\uparrow$ pH value)
9. Contamination with meconium

Cord blood sampling for pH after fetal delivery is becoming more routine, and the sample is an indicator of fetal status at the time of delivery. This is done by obtaining a sample of cord blood between double clamps on the umbilical cord. This information may be useful if questions arise as to fetal status at the time of birth.

Procedure for fetal blood sampling

The procedure for *fetal blood sampling* (Figure 7-3) requires that the membranes be ruptured and that the presenting part be accessible. The cervix must be dilated at least 2.5 cm to allow secure placement of the endoscope against the fetal head. The patient is placed in lithotomy position, and the external perineal area is prepared with an antibacterial solution. Sterile gloves should be worn and the patient prepped and draped in a sterile manner. The lateral position may be used for those patients who have supine hypotension syndrome. The presenting part is visualized with an amnioscope, a long cone-shaped instrument with an attached light source. Fetal hair may need to be parted to better expose the scalp. This area is then cleansed with a sterile cotton swab to en-

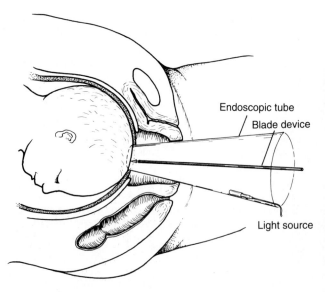

Figure 7-3
Schema of fetal blood sampling.

sure a specimen uncontaminated with amniotic fluid or mucus. Some physicians may spray the area with ethyl chloride to induce a local hyperemia. Silicone gel applied to a small sponge is inserted through the amnioscope with a sponge holder and applied to the fetal head. This promotes the beading of blood droplets. A 2 mm blade on a long handle is then inserted to make a small stab wound. Caution must be exercised to avoid puncture over the fontaneles. The heparinized glass capillary tube is held with the tip in contact with the blood, which will fill the tube by capillary action. One end of the tube is sealed and a small metal rod inserted in the other end before sealing it as well. A magnet passed over the tube mixes the blood and heparin by moving the metal rod from one end to the other. Pressure is applied to the puncture site with a sterile cotton ball—usually through the next two contractions—to ensure hemostasis. The incidence of complications such as hemorrhage and scalp abscess is less than 1%.

Interpretation of values

The normal range of pH in an adult is 7.35 to 7.45. The average fetal range is 7.30 to 7.35, with values above 7.25 considered normal. A value between 7.20 and 7.25 is considered preacidotic, and the blood sample is usually repeated within 15 to 30 minutes to detect the possibility of a downward trend. A scalp blood pH of less than 7.20 is considered frank acidosis and is indicative of the need for some type of medical or surgical intervention.

Normal Fetal Scalp Values

pH	7.25-7.35
P_{O_2}	18-22 mm Hg
P_{CO_2}	40-50 mm Hg

Base deficit approximately 7 mEq/L

Anaerobic metabolism will occur in the fetus in the absence of oxygen, resulting in the production of lactic acid, which accumulates to lower the fetal pH and thus serves as an indirect measure of fetal oxygenation. When respiratory acidosis occurs in the fetus, as can occur with cord compression demonstrated by variable decelerations, the pH is low, the P_{CO_2} markedly elevated, and the base deficit usually unchanged. With metabolic acidosis caused by uteroplacental insufficiency and demonstrated by late decelerations, the pH is low; the Po_2 decreased, the Pco_2 mildly elevated; and the base deficit elevated, possibly exceeding 10 to 15 mEq/L.

Umbilical cord acid-base determination

A useful adjunct to the Apgar score in assessing the immediate condition of the newborn is to obtain a sample of cord blood. It is as yet undetermined how useful this might be in all deliveries; however, it may be helpful to rule out asphyxia in the presence of a low Apgar score. If metabolic acidosis is not present, then it is not likely that the low Apgar score is due to intrapartum asphyxia.

The procedure consists of double clamping a 10 to 20 cm (approximately 4 to 8 inches) segment of the umbilical cord immediately after delivery of the infant. A specimen should be drawn with a 1-ml plastic syringe that has been flushed with heparin solution (1000 U/ml.), from the umbilical artery, or if that is not possible, from the umbilical vein. Residual air or heparin should be ejected from the syringe and the needle capped. The normal values are summarized as follows:

Normal Values for Umbilical Cord Blood

Cord blood	pH	Pco_2 mm Hg	Po_2 mm Hg	Bicarbonate mEq/L
Arterial	7.28	49.2	18.0	22.3
(range)	(7.15-7.43)	(31.1-74.3)	(3.8-33.8)	(13.3-27.5)
Venous	7.35	38.2	29.2	20.4
(range)	(7.24-7.49)	(23.2-49.2)	(15.4-48.2)	(15.9-24.7)

Adjuvant Treatment for Fetal Distress
Amnioinfusion

Amnioinfusion is a procedure involving the replacement of amniotic fluid with normal saline through the intrauterine pressure catheter in patients at risk for developing cord compression, as evidenced by variable decelerations, or in patients already experiencing variable decelerations during labor. The purpose is to correct oligohydramnios, which makes the umbilical cord more vulnerable to compression during uterine contractions. Amnioinfusion often relieves both the frequency and intensity of variable decelerations.

Indications

1. Laboring preterm patients with premature rupture of the membranes
2. Patients with otherwise uncorrectable variable decelerations during labor
3. Known cases of significant oligohydramnios (or meconium-stained amniotic fluid) at term when undergoing induction of labor

Equipment and supplies

1000 ml/normal saline solution (at room temperature)
1. Internal uterine catheter equipment
2. Intravenous extension tubing with twin sites or arterial line (12 inches) and a four-way stopcock
3. Volumetric infusion pump and tubing
4. Blood warmer or blood fluid warming set (optional)

NOTE: When the fetus is preterm and the procedure is being done prophylactically, a volumetric infusion pump and warming unit or normal saline warmed to body temperature (98.6° F) should be used.

Preprocedure

1. Place patient in left lateral position
2. Administer oxygen by face mask 8 to 12 L/min if ordered by the physician
3. Continuously monitor the patient

Procedure

After the intrauterine catheter is inserted and connected to the strain gauge:
1. Connect the extension tubing, which has been prefilled with sterile distilled water (to prevent saline corrosion of the transducer), between the three-way stopcock (connected to the pressure transducer) and the intrauterine catheter
2. Attach intravenous tubing to the bottle of room temperature normal saline

3. Attach the 18-gauge needle to the intravenous tubing connected to the saline
4. Insert the needle into the side port of the extension tubing just above the connection to the intrauterine catheter
5. Initiate the flow of normal saline solution and instill 15 to 20 ml/min until variable decelerations are resolved or start the infusion at 600 ml/hr (10 ml/min), then decrease to 180 ml/hr as indicated by fetal response. This can be achieved when the saline bottle is 3 to 4 feet above the level of the intrauterine catheter tip and when the intravenous control device is wide open, or this can be done by administering the solution through a volumetric infusion pump
   a. When variable decelerations diminish or resolve, add an additional 250 ml of normal saline to promote a continuing variable deceleration-free FHR pattern
   b. If variable decelerations are not relieved after infusion of 800 ml of normal saline solution, then procedure may be discontinued and alternate interventions performed

Be aware that the recorded resting tone during amnioinfusion will appear higher than normal, about 35 to 40 mm Hg because of resistance to outflow through the tiny holes in the tip of the catheter. The true resting tone can be checked easily by shutting off the infusion.

Optional setup

A 12-inch arterial line extension tubing can be used instead of the flexible type of extension tubing. Using a four-way stopcock between the intrauterine catheter and the arterial line will permit turning the infusion off to read the intrauterine pressure without any distortion from the amnioinfusion.

Patient care

Care of the patient undergoing amnioinfusion includes the following:
1. Stop the infusion periodically to note the baseline uterine pressure, approximately every 30 minutes. Notify the physician if the resting tone is greater than 25 mm Hg to evaluate continuation of the procedure
2. Change the underpads frequently to ensure patient comfort. This is necessary because of the increase in vaginal fluid leakage.

Tocolysis Therapy for Abnormal Fetal Heart Rate Patterns

Although tocolytic therapy is routinely used to prevent and manage preterm labor, it can be used as an adjunct to other interventions in the management of fetal distress. Drugs used for the preterm labor patient who is at less than 37 weeks' gestation include magnesium sulfate and beta-sympathomimetics such as terbutaline and ritodrine. When the fetus is exhibiting signs of acute distress with concomitant increased uterine activity that is not responsive to position change and discontinuance of the oxytocin infusion, the administration of an intravenous injection of terbutaline of 0.125 to 0.250 mg can be administered while preparation for immediate delivery is in process. A cesarean delivery may be performed if the abnormal FHR pattern persists and the fetus cannot be safely delivered vaginally. Conversely, if the FHR pattern improves, then the patient may be allowed to continue labor. Terbutaline, which has a shorter time of onset, is preferred to magnesium sulfate, which has a longer time of onset of 10 to 15 minutes.

NOTE: A protocol for the "Management of Preterm Labor" that describes the use of tocolytics for patients meeting the criteria for the diagnosis of preterm labor can be found in Appendix C.

Antepartum Monitoring

8

Evaluation of fetal well-being and maturity is essential in the management of high-risk pregnancy. The contraction stress test (CST), the nonstress test (NST), and fetal movement counts have been widely employed for the determination of fetal well-being.

Some indications for both the NST and the CST follow:

1. Suspected postmaturity (postdates ≥42 weeks)
2. Maternal diabetes mellitus
3. Chronic hypertension
4. Hypertensive disorders in pregnancy
5. Suspected intrauterine growth retardation
6. Sickle cell disease
7. Maternal cyanotic heart disease
8. History of previous stillbirth
9. Blood group sensitization (isoimmunization)
10. Meconium-stained amniotic fluid (at amniocentesis)
11. Hyperthyroidism
12. Collagen vascular diseases
13. Older gravida (more than 35 years)
14. Chronic renal disease
15. Decreasing (or apparently absent) fetal movement
16. Severe maternal anemia
17. Discordant twins

Nonstress Test
Description

The basis for the NST to assess fetal well-being is that the normal fetus will produce characteristic heart rate patterns. Average relative baseline variability and acceleration of FHR in response to fetal movement are reassuring signs. The FHR pattern assessed by external monitoring techniques without any stress or stimuli to the fetus.

When hypoxia, acidosis, or drugs depress the fetal central nervous system, there may be a reduction in baseline variability and absence of FHR acceleration with fetal movement. The patterns can also be produced by quiet fetal sleep states, and therefore it is sometimes necessary to monitor 20 to 30 minutes or more until the fetus is in a more active state or to palpate the abdomen to activate the resting fetus.

Indications and contraindications

The indications for the NST are the same as for the CST. There are no contraindications to the NST.

Preparation and procedure (Figure 8-1)

An advantage of the NST over the CST is that it can be performed in an outpatient setting. Prepare the patient for the NST by taking a baseline blood pressure, then applying the external mode of monitoring with the patient in semi-Fowler's position.

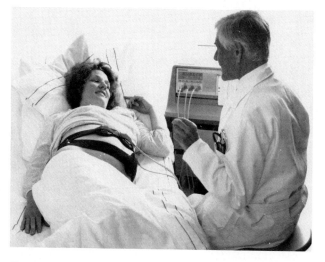

Figure 8-1
Antepartum monitoring of twin gestation (note dual ultrasound transducers).
(Courtesy Hewlett-Packard Company, Andover, Mass.)

The observer identifies fetal movement on the chart paper as evidenced by spikes or momentary increases in uterine pressure. If evidence of fetal movement is not apparent on the chart paper, the patient is asked to depress a button on a hand-held event marker that is connected into the appropriate outlet on the monitor when she feels fetal movement. The "event" of fetal movement is then noted by a spike of arrow printed by the stylus on the uterine activity (UA) panel of the monitor strip. If necessary, fetal movement can be facilitated by palpation of the abdomen to activate the resting fetus. The maternal blood pressure may be monitored during the procedure as indicated and at the end of the procedure. The procedure usually lasts 20 minutes but may need to be extended if criteria for a reactive pattern have not been met. If the pattern is questionable or if decelerations occur, the CST is then performed.

Interpretation

The following guidelines for evaluation of the NST are offered, although minor variations in criteria are successfully used by various institutions:

Reactive test (Figure 8-2)	Two or more FHR accelerations of at least 15 bpm lasting at least 15 seconds in a 20-minute period; baseline rate is within the normal range, and variability is average
Nonreactive test (Figure 8-3)	Absence of accelerations of FHR during the testing period
Inconclusive test	Less than one acceleration in a 20-minute period or one that is less than 15 bpm and lasts less than 15 seconds; variability less than 6 bpm or quality of FHR recording not adequate for interpretation

Clinical significance and management

The reactive test suggests that the fetus would be born in good condition were labor to occur in a few days. However, when the NST is used for primary fetal surveillance, it should be performed semiweekly in high-risk patients, especially those with postdate pregnancies and diabetes or IUGR. As long as twice-weekly NSTs remain reactive, most high-risk pregnancies are allowed to continue. The nonreactive test should be followed as soon as possible by a contraction stress test (CST). Those pa-

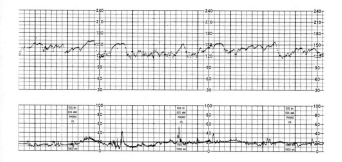

Figure 8-2
Reactive nonstress test (FHR acceleration with fetal movement).

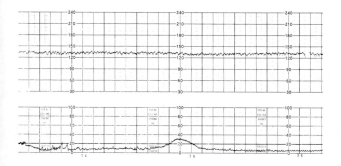

Figure 8-3
Nonreactive nonstress test (no FHR acceleration with fetal movement).

tients with an inconclusive test may have the NST repeated in several hours, or may have a CST or biophysical profile (BPP), according to the clinical assessment of the physician.

Inasmuch as a nonreactive or inconclusive test can be caused by fetal sleep states, an attempt should be made to stimulate the fetus by manipulating the uterus and continuing to monitor the fetus for another 20- or 30-minute period.

Acoustic Stimulation

The acoustic stimulation test is another method of testing FHR response. The test takes a short time to complete, and the procedure is as follows:

1. Monitor the FHR and uterine activity until at least 10 minutes of interpretable data are obtained. If there are no spontaneous accelerations of FHR, then proceed to the next step.
2. Apply the artificial larynx or a fetal acoustic stimulation device firmly to the maternal abdomen over the fetal head.
3. Depress the button on the device for a single 1- to 2-second sound stimulation. (At the same time it is preferable to depress the event marker, which will mark the uterine activity panel of the monitor strip.)
4. Observe and document the FHR response.
5. Repeat the stimulus at 1-minute intervals up to three times if FHR accelerations do not occur after the first acoustic stimulus.

Interpretation

Reactive Test: Two FHR accelerations of 15 bpm for 15 seconds in response to acoustic stimulation within 10 minutes
Nonreactive Test: Inability to fulfill the criterion for reactivity as described above within 10 minutes

Clinical significance and management

Because most authors refer to acoustic stimulation as a modified nonstress test, the clinical significance is the same as that of the NST. Management of the patient with a reactive test includes ongoing surveillance. Those with a nonreactive test should have a contraction stress test (CST) performed and a biophysical profile, or both.

Contraction Stress Test

The basis for the CST is that a healthy fetus can withstand a decreased oxygen supply during the physiological stress of a contraction, whereas a compromised fetus will demonstrate late decelerations that are nonreassuring and indicative of uteroplacental insufficiency.

CSTs can be performed with endogenously produced oxytocin as stimulated by breast and nipple manipulation, or the test can be performed with an exogenous source of oxytocin administered by intravenous infusion.

Although the NST can be performed on any patient, the CST cannot. The potential for preterm labor precludes performing the test on patients with certain high-risk conditions.

The CST is contraindicated in the following situations:

1. Premature rupture of membranes
2. Placenta previa
3. Third trimester bleeding
4. Previous classical cesarean section
5. Multiple gestation
6. Incompetent cervix
7. Hydramnios
8. History of preterm labor

The two types of CST are the nipple-stimulated contraction stress test and the oxytocin challenge test.

Nipple-stimulated contraction stress test

Procedure	Rationale
1. Assist the patient to a semi-Fowler's position	1. To avoid supine hypotension
2. Place the tocotransducer where the least maternal tissue is in evidence, usually above the umbilicus	2. To ensure that the fundus is as close as possible to the pressure sensing device
3. Place the ultrasound transducer on the maternal abdomen where the clearest fetal signal can be obtained	3. To ensure that the tracing is clear and interpretable

Procedure	Rationale
4. Monitor baseline FHR and uterine activity until 10 minutes of interpretable data are obtained (defer nipple stimulation if three spontaneous unstimulated contractions of more than 40 seconds duration occur within a 10-minute period)	4. To provide a basis for comparison (it may not be necessary to proceed with test if spontaneous contractions occur)
5. Instruct patient to brush palmar surface of the fingers over the nipple of one breast through her clothes; continue 4 cycles of 2 minutes on and 2 minutes off; stop when contraction begins and restimulate when contraction ends (if a 2 minute period has elapsed)	5. To stimulate oxytocin secretion into the circulation from the pituitary gland
a. If unsuccessful after 4 cycles, restimulate the breasts for 10 minutes, stopping when contraction begins and resuming when contraction ends	a. To maintain uterine contractions
b. If unsuccessful, begin bilateral continuous stimulation for 10 minutes, stopping when contraction begins and resuming when contraction ends	
6. Discontinue nipple stimulation when 3 or more spontaneous contractions lasting longer than 40 seconds occur in a 10-minute period and are palpable to the examiner	6. To eliminate unnecessary stress

Procedure	Rationale
7. Interpret results and continue monitoring until uterine activity has returned to the prestimulation state	7. To ensure that the patient and fetus are restored to their prestress status

If nipple stimulation does not produce the desired uterine activity, an oxytocin-stimulated CST is indicated. Interpretation guidelines for contraction stress testing are described after the oxytocin challenge test (OCT).

Oxytocin challenge test

The OCT is routinely performed in the inpatient setting, since labor may be stimulated in some sensitive patients, particularly in those at term.

Procedure	Rationale
1. Assist patient into a semi-Fowler's position	1. To avoid supine hypotension
2. Place the tocotransducer where the least maternal tissue is in evidence, usually above the umbilicus	2. To ensure that the fundus is as close as possible to the pressure-sensing button
3. Place the ultrasound transducer where the clearest fetal heart sound can be heard, usually below the umbilicus	3. To obtain a clear fetal signal
4. Monitor baseline FHR and uterine activity until 10 minutes of interpretable data are obtained before administration of oxytocin	4. To provide a basis for comparison
5. Check the patient's blood pressure and pulse every 10 to 15 minutes	5. To identify hypotension resulting from maternal position

Procedure	Rationale
6. If less than three spontaneous unstimulated contractions occur within a 10-minute period and if late decelerations do not occur with spontaneous contractions, oxytocin can be initiated	6. Oxytocin stimulation may not be necessary if adequate uterine activity is present; test may be discontinued if late decelerations occur with spontaneous contractions
7. Piggyback oxytocin into the primary IV line (with lactated Ringer's or other nonaqueous solution)	7. May be necessary to rapidly infuse the primary IV in the event of uterine hyperstimulation or maternal hypotension
8. Administer oxytocin beginning with 0.25 mU/ minute with a constant infusion pump	8. To ensure specific dosage of oxytocin
9. Increase the dosage of oxytocin infusion by 0.5 mU/minute at 15-minute intervals until the contraction frequency is three in 10 minutes of 40 to 60 seconds duration and contractions are palpable to the examiner	9. To ensure a safe rate of oxytocin increments; generally the dosage of oxytocin does not exceed 5 mU/ minute, but occasional doses of up to 10 mU/ minute may be necessary
10. Discontinue the oxytocin when three contractions have occurred within a 10-minute period of interpretable data	10. To provide an adequate stress from which an interpretation can be made
11. Discontinue the oxytocin anytime there is evidence of hyperstimulation, prolonged bradycardia, or consistent late decelerations; treat fetal distress in the same manner as during intrapartum monitoring	11. To prevent additional fetal distress; the principles for treating fetal distress apply during both antepartum and intrapartum monitoring

Procedure	Rationale
12. Continue to monitor until uterine activity and FHR return to baseline status	12. To ensure that the patient and fetus are restored to their prestress status

Interpretation

1. Negative test (Figure 8-4)	1. Three uterine contractions in a 10-minute period without late decelerations; there is usually average baseline variability and acceleration of FHR with fetal movement
2. Positive test (Figure 8-5)	2. Persistent late decelerations or late decelerations with more than half the contractions; may be associated with minimal or absent variability
3. Suspicious test	3. Late decelerations occurring with less than half the uterine contractions
4. Hyperstimulation	4. Contractions occurring more often than every 2 minutes or lasting longer than 90 seconds, or if there is apparent hypertonus associated with contractions; if no late decelerations occur with the preceding, the test is interpreted as negative; if late deceleration is observed during or after excessive uterine activity, the test is not interpretable and is classified as hyperstimulation because the stress is considered enough to exceed even normal uteroplacental reserve
5. Unsatisfactory	5. Quality of the recording is not sufficient to be sure that no late decelerations are present or where less than three uterine contractions have occurred in a 10-minute period; the test is not interpretable and cannot be used for clinical management

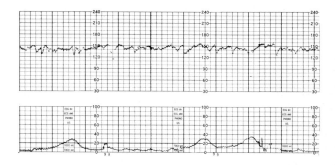

Figure 8-4
Negative contraction stress test (reassuring external tracing).

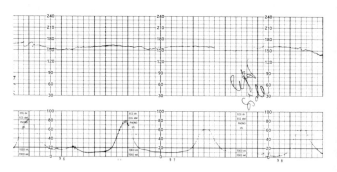

Figure 8-5
Positive contraction stress test (late decelerations with uterine contractions).

The CST is highly reliable when it is negative, and false negatives are very rare. On the other hand, false positives occur when there are FHR accelerations with fetal movement. In contrast, when there is an absence of late decelerations in a patient in labor with a previous positive CST, it may be indicative of a correction of uteroplacental insufficiency in the interval between the test and labor and not a false positive CST.

Clinical significance and management

A negative CST is reassuring that the fetus is likely to survive labor should it occur within 1 week, as long as there is no change in status of either the mother or the fetus. This may permit a postponement of intervention until fetal lung maturity is achieved. As an indicator of fetoplacental respiratory reserve the CST cannot preclude fetal death from obstetrical emergencies such as abruptio placentae and prolapsed cord. Preterm labor is not associated with a CST. If the fetus is less than 38 weeks' gestation, labor almost never begins within 48 hours after the procedure.

False positives can occur when FHR accelerations with fetal movement are observed. Therefore management of the patient with a positive CST is not as clear cut. It lies somewhere between fetal assessment with other techniques and immediate termination of pregnancy. There is, of course, no substitute for expert clinical judgment as to the course of action to be taken.

CSTs resulting in hyperstimulation or suspicious or unsatisfactory results are repeated in 24 hours. If interpretable data cannot be achieved, other methods of fetal assessment must be used.

Fetal Movement

Various investigators have reported a marked decrease in fetal movement before an episode of fetal distress or fetal death. It is interesting to note that now there is scientific evidence for a concept believed, practiced, and relied on by generations of midwives and mothers.

Daily fetal movement count (DFMC) has been studied in various ways. Mothers have recorded all fetal movements from 9 AM to 9 PM in one study and in another reclined in the left lateral position for 10 minutes three times a day, counting fetal movements occurring during those periods. As measured by an electromagnetic device, varying percentages of fetal movements were perceived by the mothers.

Generally, the number of fetal movements decreases from early to late pregnancy in normal gestation. In pregnancies complicated by uteroplacental insufficiency, there was a marked decrease in DFMC, and a precipitous fall occurred in the period immediately preceding fetal death. The advantages of this "test" are that it is inexpensive, continuously available away from the clinical area, and relatively simple for the patient to do, although accuracy and reliability are variable.

Should a patient complain of decreased fetal movement, she may be asked by the physician to lie down for 1 hour and count all the fetal movements. If she feels three or more during that time, she can be reassured. However, she should continue to be aware of fetal movements and report the hourly observations should the problem recur. An NST is often performed if only one or two movements are felt within a 1-hour period. If the NST is reactive, no further testing is done unless there are some other risk factors. A nonreactive NST would be followed as soon as possible by a CST, the potential outcomes and significance of which have been previously described.

Biophysical Profile
Description

A physical examination of the fetus using real-time ultrasound equipment. Parameters measured in this evaluation include:
1. Fetal breathing movements (FBM)
2. Fetal movement (FM)
3. Fetal tone (FT)
4. Amniotic fluid index (AFI)
5. Nonstress test (NST)

Interpretation
Biophysical profile scoring

Biophysical Variable	Normal (Score = 2)	Abnormal (Score = 0)
Fetal breathing movements	At least one episode of FBM of at least 30 sec duration in 30-min observation	Absent FBM or no episode of ≥30 sec in 30 min
Gross body movements	At least three discrete body/limb movements in 30 min (episodes of active continuous movement considered as a single movement)	Two or fewer episodes of body/limb movements in 30 min
Fetal tone	At least one episode of active extension with return to flexion of fetal limb(s) or trunk. Opening and closing of hand considered normal tone	Either slow extension with return to partial flexion or movement of limb in full extension or absence of fetal movement
Amniotic fluid index	One or more pockets of fluid measuring ≥1 cm in two perpendicular planes	Either no pockets or a pocket <1 cm in two perpendicular planes
Nonstress test	Reactive—two or more episodes of FHR acceleration ≥15 bpm ≥15 sec	Nonreactive

The Biophysical Profile should be recorded on the patient's progress sheet.

Parameter	Score
Fetal Breathing Movements (FBM)	
Fetal Movement (FM)	
Fetal Tone (FT)	
Amniotic Fluid Index (AFI)	
Nonstress Test (NST)	

TOTAL:_____

Management

Score	Action
8-10	Equivalent to reactive NST; manage per protocol
4-6	If pulmonary maturity is favorable, deliver; if not, repeat test in 24 hours; if score persists, deliver if maturity is certain; otherwise, treat with corticosteroids to promote pulmonary maturity and deliver in 48 hours
0-2	Evaluate for delivery

Home Uterine Activity Monitoring for Patients at Risk of Preterm Delivery

A lightweight tocodynamometer designed for ambulatory home monitoring, data storage, and telephone transmission of uterine activity has been developed and is in limited use for the purpose of detecting uterine activity in patients at risk for preterm labor. Patients using this device are given detailed instructions regarding frequency of self-monitoring and asked to phone a study center daily to transmit the data. Those with four or more contractions an hour are usually referred for in-hospital monitoring. In addition to patients at risk for preterm labor, the device has been used on those whose preterm labor was arrested with parenteral tocolytics and who continue to take oral tocolytics at home.

This modality has the potential of reducing the preterm birth rate, and further studies will determine its efficiency in terms of home monitoring for high-risk pregnancy management.

Care of the Monitored Patient

9

The care given to the monitored patient in labor is the same care given to any patient during labor, with additional consideration to those factors that relate directly to the monitor. The most important item by far is a thorough explanation to the patient and her labor coach (usually her husband) about the fetal monitor—how it is used and how it is applied. Many patients are anxious about the status of the baby, concluding that something must be wrong for the monitor to be used. Some patients fear the machine itself and are distracted by its mechanical noises and beeps. Others are afraid to move in bed for fear of dislodging the leads and are concerned that the leads can harm the baby. The digital display of FHR is also frequently a source of anxiety. Because it cannot print out every heartbeat, a sampling of FHR is displayed, and often very low or very high numbers are observed. Patients expressing concern over those numbers should be told that the main reason for the digital display is not to demonstrate the actual FHR but to assist in testing the instrument, and that variations in the displayed FHR are expected. Patient acceptance of the monitor can usually be gained by a thorough explanation of the factors causing the patient's anxiety.

In contrast, the monitor is often reassuring to the patient. An audible "beep" of the fetal heart sounds can be reassuring that all is well with the fetus. This sound often serves as encouragement to the patient, especially during late labor when some patients, distracted by their discomfort, lose sight of the reason for it, momentarily forgetting about the imminent birth of their baby. For those patients who feel as if they will be "pregnant forever," it is often reassuring to see evidence of uterine contractions on the strip chart paper.

There is usually no contraindication to showing the patient and her labor coach the monitor strip differentiating FHR from uterine activity. Even when this is not shown to them, they quickly identify and contrast the FHR from the uterine activity (UA) panel without much difficulty. Patients do observe changes in the monitoring pattern, such as those caused by fetal movement, and can be given appropriate explanations when decelerations or dips in the FHR occur. After all, in an emergency situation such as a prolapsed umbilical cord, when the examiner's fingers are manually supporting the presenting part away from the cord until a cesarean section can be done, there are no real secrets about the urgency of the situation.

Care of the electronically monitored patient in labor is the same as care of the patient in labor who is not electronically monitored. One needs to be certain that the monitor does not receive more attention than the patient. However, the patient who is monitored should receive additional personal attention because of the mode of monitoring used. Guidelines for care are described in the following quick-reference outline format:

Care of the Patient on a Fetal Monitor

Observations

Patient's position

Patient's comfort

Respiratory rate and pattern

Temperature

Blood pressure

Voiding pattern

Uterine contraction pattern;
   frequency, duration, intensity, resting tone

Fetal heart rate, baseline rate, variability, accelerations, decelerations

Placement and functioning of external transducers (tocotransducer, ultrasound transducer) and internal devices (spiral electrode, intrauterine pressure catheter)

Adjustment of equipment

Cervical effacement and dilatation

Fetal presentation and position

Status of membranes

Color and amount of amniotic fluid

Ongoing care

Test monitor on initiation and as needed

Position patient comfortably

Encourage lateral position if bed is flat (modify this if patient is in semi-Fowler's position) to prevent supine hypotension syndrome

Chart all nursing and patient care activities on monitor strip

During the first stage of labor:

Document FHR q15 to 30 min (in low-risk patients)

When risk factors are present, document FHR q15 min when intermittent auscultation is used;

if the patient is electronically monitored, the strip chart should be evaluated q15 min and initialed to verify this

During the second stage of labor

Evaluate and record the FHR q5 min when auscultation is used in patients with risk factors

Evaluate the FHR strip chart on electronically monitored patients with risk factors q5 min

In low-risk patients the FHR should be documented q15 min (if auscultated) or the strip chart reviewed, evaluated, and initialed for patients who are electronically monitored

Document FHR immediately after membranes rupture and again in 5 min

(Table 9-1)

Table 9-1   Fetal monitoring equipment checklist

| Name: _____ | Evaluator: _____ | | |
| Date: _____ | | | |
Items to be Checked	Yes	No	Remarks
Preparation of Monitor			
1. Is the paper inserted correctly?			
2. Are transducer cables plugged into appropriate outlet of the monitor?			

Continued.

Table 9-1   Fetal monitoring equipment checklist—cont'd

Name: _____   Evaluator: _____

Date: _____

Items to be Checked	Yes	No	Remarks
Ultrasound Transducer			
1. Has transmission gel been applied to the ultrasound?			
2. Was the FHR tested and noted on the monitor strip?			
3. Does a signal light flash with each heartbeat?			
4. Is the strap secure and snug?			
Tocotransducer			
1. Is the tocotransducer firmly strapped where the least maternal tissue is in evidence?			
2. Has it been applied without gel or paste?			
3. Was the penset knob adjusted between 20 and 25 mm marks and noted on chart paper?			
4. Was this setting done between contractions?			
5. Is the strap secure and snug?			
Spiral Electrode			
1. Are the wires attached firmly to the posts on the leg plate?			
2. Is the spiral electrode attached to the presenting part of the fetus?			
3. Is the inner surface of the leg plate covered with electrode paste (if necessary)?			
4. Is the leg plate properly secured to the patient's thigh?			

Table 9-1   Fetal monitoring equipment checklist—cont'd

| Name: _____ | Evaluator: _____ | | |
| Date: _____ | | | |

Items to be Checked	Yes	No	Remarks
Internal Catheter			
1. Is the length line on the catheter visible at the introitus?			
2. Is it noted on the chart paper that a calibration was done?			
3. Was the uterine activity tested?			

External Monitoring
Ultrasound transducer

(Monitors FHR with high-frequency sound waves)

Tap transducer before use to ensure sound transmission

Apply ultrasound transmission gel to maternal abdomen

Clean abdomen and transducer and reapply gel prn

Massage reddened skin areas and reposition belt prn

Auscultate FHR with stethoscope or fetoscope if in doubt as to the validity of monitor strip

Position and reposition transducer as needed to ensure clear interpretable FHR data

Tocotransducer

(Monitors uterine activity via a pressure-sensing device placed on the maternal abdomen)

Position and reposition as needed on the fundus where the least maternal tissue is in evidence

Maintain snug abdominal strap

Adjust penset *between* contractions to print between 20 and 25 mm Hg on the monitor strip

Palpate fundus every 30 to 60 minutes to gauge strength of contraction; only frequency and duration of contractions can be assessed with tocotransducer

Do not assess patient's need for analgesic based on uterine activity displayed on strip chart

Massage reddened areas under transducer and belt and relocate qh and prn

Internal Monitoring
Spiral electrode

(Obtains fetal ECG from presenting part and converts to FHR)

Ensure that color-coded wires are appropriately attached to push post on leg plate if indicated

Apply electrode paste to leg plate prn

Observe FHR panel of strip chart for long- and short-term variability

Turn electrode counterclockwise to remove; *never* pull straight out from presenting part

Administer perineal care after voiding and prn

Intrauterine catheter

(Fluid-filled catheter internally monitors intrauterine pressure)

Ensure that length line on catheter is visible at introitus

For fluid-filled catheters, turn stopcock off to patient, release pressure valve of strain gauge, flush strain gauge, remove syringe, and set printer to 0 line on monitor paper; test further as needed, according to manufacturer's instructions

Check proper functioning by tapping catheter, asking patient to cough, or applying fundal pressure; observe appropriate inflection on monitor strip

Keep catheter taped to patient's leg to prevent dislodgment

 Patient Teaching

Ensure that the patient and her significant other know and understand that the:

Use of the monitor does not imply fetal jeopardy

Fetal status via FHR can be continuously assessed even during contractions

Lower panel on the strip chart shows uterine activity and that the upper panel shows FHR

Prepared childbirth techniques can be implemented without difficulty

Effleurage performed during external monitoring can be done on the sides of the abdomen or upper thighs

Breathing patterns based on timing and intensity of contraction can be enhanced by observation of the uterine activity panel of the strip chart for onset of contractions

Note peak of contraction; knowing that contraction will not get stronger and is half over is usually helpful

Note diminishing intensity

Coordinate with appropriate breathing and relaxation techniques

Use of internal mode of monitoring does not restrict patient movement

Use of external mode of monitoring usually requires patient cooperation is positioning and movement

Documentation

The adage "if it was not documented, then it was not done" clearly applies to fetal monitoring and care of the patient in labor, especially when this information may be reviewed months or years later in legal action. It is imperative to have excellent records. Information that should be included on the monitor strip beginning, during, and after monitoring follows:

1. Beginning of monitoring
   a. Patient's name and age
   b. Identification number
   c. Date
   d. Physician's name
   e. Time the monitor was attached and mode
   f. Testing/calibration
   g. Gravida _____ Para _____
   h. Expected date of confinement (EDC)
   i. Monitor code number
   j. High-risk factors (e.g., pregnancy-induced hypertension, diabetes)
   k. Membranes intact or ruptured
   l. Gestational age
   m. Dilatation and station
2. During the course of monitoring
   a. Maternal position and repositioning in bed
   b. Vaginal examination and results
   c. Analgesia or anesthesia
   d. Medication given
   e. BP, T, P, and R
   f. Voidings
   g. O_2 given

    h. Emesis
    i. Pushing
    j. Fetal movement
    k. Any change in mode of monitoring
    l. Adjustments of equipment
       (1) Relocation of transducers
       (2) Adjustment or flushing of catheter
       (3) Replacement of electrode
       (4) Replacement or removal of catheter
    m. Intervention for nonreassuring FHR patterns
    n. Signature and time the strip is evaluated (according to hospital policy, usually every 30 minutes or less)

        This procedure ensures that someone has assessed the patient and FHR on a regular basis and ensures that a nonreassuring pattern is observed and subsequently treated.

        These notations are important for retrospective audit and teaching purposes and they are of the utmost importance in identifying the cause of a specific FHR response to nursing or medical action.

3. On completion of monitoring and delivery, the nurse should make the following summary notations at the end of the chart paper:
    a. Delivery date and time
    b. Type of delivery
    c. Anesthesia
    d. Sex and weight of the infant
    e. Presentation
    f. Both 1- and 5-minute Apgar scores
    g. Complications
    h. Presence or absence of meconium
    i. Cord blood pH, if done

The monitor strip then presents a complete picture of the patient's labor.

Pattern Interpretation

Interpretation of the FHR pattern and uterine activity should be done in a thorough, systematic fashion. The baseline FHR should be identified as being within the normal fetal heart range, tachycardia, or bradycardia. The degree of baseline variability should be assessed, noting the presence or absence of short- and long-term variability. Periodic changes should be noted as accelerations of FHR and early, late, or variable decelerations. Uterine activity should be assessed by the frequency and duration of contractions, and if the patient is monitored internally, the intensity and resting tone of the uterus in millimeters of mercury pressure can be identified. A tool for assessment of the fetal monitor strip chart is offered in Table 9-2 and can be used when monitoring is in progress or after delivery for audit or teaching purposes.

The significance of appropriate use of equipment and assessment of the FHR monitor strip cannot be overemphasized. Individuals caring for patients sometimes have the opportunity to review their documentation during legal proceedings. The prudent caretaker will ensure that all equipment is appropriately used and that patient care activities, including assessment and interventions, are appropriate and documented in a clear, concise, and objective manner.

Table 9-2   Fetal heart rate assessment checklist

Patient's Name _____ Date/Time _____

1. What is the baseline fetal heart rate (FHR)?
   _____ Beats per minute (bpm)
   Check one of the following as observed on the monitor strip:
   _____ Average baseline FHR (120 to 160 bpm)
   _____ Tachycardia (>120 bpm or >30 bpm from normal/
   previous baseline)
   _____ Bradycardia (<120 bpm or <30 bpm from normal/
   previous baseline)
2. What is the baseline variability?
   _____ Average short-term variability (6 to 10 bpm)
   _____ Average long-term variability (3 to 5 cycles per
   minute)
   _____ Minimal variability
   _____ Absence of variability
   _____ Marked variability

Continued.

Table 9-2   Fetal heart rate assessment checklist—cont'd

Patient's Name _____ Date/Time _____

3. Are there any periodic changes in FHR?
   _____ Accelerations with fetal movement
   _____ Repetitive accelerations with each contraction
   _____ Early decelerations (head compression)
   _____ Late decelerations (uteroplacental insufficiency)
   Variable decelerations (cord compression)
   _____ Mild
   _____ Moderate
   _____ Severe
4. What does the uterine activity panel show?
   _____ Frequency (peak to peak)
   _____ Duration (beginning to end)
   _____ Intensity (in mm Hg only with intrauterine catheter)
   _____ Resting time at least 30 seconds
   _____ Resting tone (<15 mm Hg pressure)
COMMENTS:_____

PANEL NUMBER	WHAT CAN BE OR SHOULD HAVE BEEN DONE

Professional Issues

10

Legal Aspects

The nurse is legally responsible for performing fetal monitoring according to the established standard of care as defined by the nurse's employer and the nurse's professional education, medical practice, professional organizations, and the local state nurse practice act. Observations, evaluation, and intervention for the patient's symptoms, progress, and reactions are the nurse's responsibility within legally sanctioned confines. The nurse who develops expertise in monitoring and pattern recognition is held responsible for this expertise. It is appropriate to use the terms that have been given to fetal monitoring patterns (eg., acceleration and early, late, or variable decelerations) in documentation on the patient's medical record and in verbal communication. After identification of a nonreassuring pattern the nurse's responsibility does not cease with nursing intervention alone. The attending physician must be notified and must respond to the emergency. Should the physician be unfamiliar with monitoring or have differences in interpretation, the nurse must follow hospital protocol for resolving the conflict. In most facilities the nursing supervisor is notified, who in turn confers with the medical director or chief of the obstetrical unit. It is certainly preferable to go through the appropriate chain of command than to avoid the stress of confrontation, because the alternatives of fetal deterioration and probable subsequent litigation are clearly undesirable.

The importance of documentation on the patient's record cannot be overemphasized. Adherence to standards of practice is essential, and appropriate assessment, intervention, and evaluation should be clearly documented. It behooves the practitioner to anticipate how the patient's records might be analyzed by others years after a delivery, as occurs during the litigation process. The general assumption is that what is not written did not occur, and the concept of what the reasonable, prudent nurse would do in the same situation takes on new meaning to those who become involved in medical malpractice.

Increasing concern for competency in fetal monitoring has stimulated discussion and emphasized a trend toward the need for validating that competency (such as by a written certification examination). Electronic FHR monitoring is but one method of fetal assessment and cannot conceptually, or practically, be separated from other clinical assessment techniques or from the normal, high-risk, and pathophysiological processes that occur during the antepartum and intrapartum periods.

With the intent of promoting competency in clinical nursing practice NAACOG has developed *Electronic Fetal Monitoring: Nursing Practice Competencies and Educational Guidelines*. The guidelines (see Appendix A) describe minimal educational preparation to achieve competency in electronic fetal monitoring and are an excellent resource for the practicing nurse, nurse manager, or administrator, as well as the nursing educator.

Glossary of Terms and Abbreviations

abruptio placentae   premature separation of the placenta before delivery of the fetus.

acceleration   transient increase in the fetal heart rate.

acidosis   a pathological condition marked by an increased concentration of hydrogen ions in tissue.

AFI   amniotic fluid index.

amniocentesis   procedure in which amniotic fluid is removed from the uterine cavity by insertion of a needle through the abdominal and uterine walls into the amniotic sac.

amnioinfusion   replacement of amniotic fluid with normal saline through an intrauterine pressure catheter.

amnion   inner of the two fetal membranes forming the sac that encloses the fetus within the uterus.

amniotomy   artificial rupture of the amniotic sac.

anencephaly   absence of the cerebrum, cerebellum, and flat bones of the skull.

angiography   x-ray examination of blood vessels made radiopaque by the injection of a radiopaque substance.

antepartum   occurring before birth.

Apgar score   quantitative estimate of the condition of an infant at 1 and 5 minutes after birth, derived by assigning points to the quality of heart rate, respiratory effort, color, muscle tone, and response to stimulation; expressed as the sum of these points with the maximum, or best, score being 10.

AROM   artificial rupture of membranes.

artifact   irregularities on a fetal monitor tracing caused by electrical interference or poor reception of the fetal heart rate signal; may appear as scattered dots or lines.

ASAP   as soon as possible.

asphyxia   condition in which there is hypoxia and metabolic acidosis.

AST   acoustic stimulation test.

atelectasis   collapse of the alveoli, or air sacs, of the lungs.

baroceptor   a pressure receptor; a nerve ending located in the walls of the carotid sinus and the aortic arch that is sensitive to stretching induced by changes in blood pressure.

baseline FHR   range of FHR present between periodic changes over a 10-minute period.

bilirubin   pigment produced by the breakdown of hemoglobin in cell elements and in red blood cells.

biparietal diameter   distance from one parietal eminence to another; can be measured by ultrasound to determine gestational age.

BP   blood pressure.

bpm   beats per minute.

bradycardia   baseline FHR below 120 bpm for 10 minutes.

CC   cord compression.

C/C/+1   used to indicate results of vaginal exam, e.g., cervix completely effaced/completely dilated/+ 1 station.

cephalopelvic disproportion (CPD)   disparity between the size of the fetal head and the maternal pelvis, preventing vaginal delivery.

chemoceptor   sensory end organ capable of reacting to a chemical stimulus.

chorion   outer of the two membranes forming the sac that encloses the fetus within the uterus.

chromosome   A dark stained body within the cell nucleus that carries hereditary factors (genes). There are 46 chromosomes in each cell except in the mature ovum and sperm, where that number is halved.

circumvallate placenta   placenta in which an overgrowth of the decidua separates the placental margin from the chorionic plate, producing a thick, white ring around the circumference of the placenta and a reduction in distribution of fetal blood vessels to the placental periphery.

cm   centimeter.

CNS   central nervous system.

CST   contraction stress test.

d/c or D/C   discontinue(d).

deceleration   a drop in the FHR; usually occurs in response to a uterine contraction.

DIL   cervical dilatation.

Doppler ultrasound   type of ultrasound that is reflected from moving interfaces such as closure of fetal heart valves. Doppler ultrasound is used in electronic fetal heart rate monitors.

DR   delivery room.

ECG   electrocardiogram.

EFF   effacement of the cervix.

effleurage   gentle stroking of the abdomen; used during labor in the Lamaze method of prepared childbirth.

EFM   electronic fetal monitor(ing).

epidural area situated on or over the dura mater. Regional anesthetic is often injected into the peridural (epidural) space of the spinal cord.

FBM fetal breathing movements.

FECG fetal electrocardiogram.

FHT fetal heart tones.

FHR fetal heart rate.

FM fetal movement.

frequency (of contractions) time from the onset of one contraction to the onset of the next or peak of one UC to the peak of the next.

FT fetal tone.

gestation pregnancy; the period of intrauterine fetal development from conception to birth.

gestational age age of a conceptus computed from the first day of the last menstrual period to any point in time thereafter.

gtt drops.

HC head compression.

HR heart rate.

hydramnios excessive volume of amniotic fluid, usually greater than 1.2 L. It is frequently seen in diabetic pregnancies and in fetuses with open neural tube defects.

hydrocephaly increased accumulation of cerebrospinal fluid within the ventricles of the brain; may result from congenital anomalies, infection, injury, or brain tumor. The head is usually large and globular with a disproportionately small face. The increased head diameter is possible in the fetus and infant because the sutures of the skull have not closed.

hydrostatic pressure pressure created in a fluid system.

hyperthermia hyperpyrexia; high fever.

hypertonic solution with a high osmotic pressure.

hypertonus excessive muscular tonus or tension.

hypothermia subnormal temperature of the body.

hypotonic solution with a low osmotic pressure.

hypoxia oxygen deficiency.

intervillous space space between the myometrium and placental villi, which is filled with maternal blood.

intrapartum occurring during labor or delivery.

IUP intrauterine pressure.

IUPC intrauterine pressure catheter.

IV intravenous (parenteral fluids).

L liter.

macrosomia large body size as seen in some postmature infants and in those born to diabetic mothers.

MECG maternal electrocardiogram.

meconium pasty greenish mass that collects in the fetal intestine, usually expelled during the first 3 to 4 days after birth. Its presence in amniotic fluid is abnormal and is usually considered a sign of fetal distress.

meningomyelocele   protrusion of a portion of the spinal cord and membranes through a defect in the vertebral column.

MHR   maternal heart rate.

min   minutes.

mm Hg   millimeters of mercury (unit of measure of pressure).

morbidity   state of being diseased or sick; the number of sick persons or cases of disease in relationship to a specific population.

mortality   the death rate; the ratio of number of deaths to a given population.

mU   milliunits (unit of oxytocin dosage).

nadir   the lowest point of a curve or FHR deceleration.

NST   nonstress test.

nuchal   neck (as in umbilical cord around the fetal neck).

OCT   oxytocin challenge test.

osmolality   quantity of a solute existing in solution as molecules or ions or both; the concentration of a solution.

osmotic pressure   pressure developed when two solutions of different concentrations of the same solute are separated by a membrane permeable to the solvent only.

PAC   premature atrial contraction.

PCB   paracervical block anesthesia.

PE   pelvic exam.

periodic changes   change in the FHR from the baseline that occurs intermittently.

piezoelectric   a substance that has the ability to convert energy from one form into another, such as mechanical pressure into electrical energy and vice versa, as with the ultrasound transducer.

PIH   pregnancy-induced hypertension.

Pit   Pitocin (oxytocin).

placenta previa   placenta covering the internal cervical os.

polyhydramnios   *see* **hydramnios.**

prn   as necessary.

PROM   premature rupture of membranes.

PVC   premature ventricular contraction.

q   every.

resting tone   intrauterine pressure between contractions (tonus).

R/O   rule out, consider as a possibility.

ROM   rupture of membranes.

sec   seconds.

sinusoidal HR pattern   baseline FHR that has a predominance of long-term variability with a characteristic sine wave pattern.

spina bifida   congenital defect in the closure of the vertebral canal with a herniated protrusion of the meninges of the cord.

spinal anesthesia   anesthesia produced by the injection of an anesthetic into the spinal subarachnoid space.

SROM   spontaneous rupture of membranes.

STA   station.

surfactant   phospholipid that normally lines the alveolar sacs after 34 weeks' gestation. Its presence prevents collapse (atelectasis) of the alveoli by permitting a small amount of air to remain in the alveoli on exhalation. The L/S ratio as measured in amniotic fluid tests for the presence of surfactant. Neonates born without surfactant develop respiratory distress syndrome (RDS).

tachycardia   baseline FHR above 160 bpm for 10 minutes.

tachysystole   excessive uterine contraction frequency.

tetany   state of increased neuromuscular irritability or spasm.

toco   tocotransducer or tocodynamometer, external device used to record uterine activity.

tocodynamometer   pressure-sensing instrument for measuring the duration and frequency of uterine contractions.

tocolytics   drugs used to inhibit uterine contractions and stop labor.

tocotransducer   *see* **tocodynamometer.**

tonus   intrauterine pressure between contractions (resting tone).

transducer   device that converts energy from one form to another; sound or pressure can be converted into an electrical impulse and vice versa.

UA   uterine activity.

UC   uterine contraction.

ultrasound transducer.   instrument that uses high-frequency sound (ultrasound) to detect moving interfaces, such as the closure of fetal heart valves, to monitor the fetal heart rate.

UPI   uteroplacental insufficiency.

US   ultrasound.

variability   fluctuations in the baseline FHR.

VBAC   vaginal birth after cesarean.

VE   vaginal exam.

Appendix A

Nursing Practice Competencies and Educational Guidelines: Antepartum Fetal Surveillance and Intrapartum Fetal Heart Monitoring

NAACOG: The Organization for Obstetric, Gynecologic and Neonatal Nurses, 409 12th Street SW, Washington, DC 20024-21

This document outlines specific areas of competency expected of each nurse whose practice includes the use of fetal surveillance techniques in assessing, promoting, and evaluating maternal and fetal well-being during the antepartum and intrapartum periods. This document also provides guidelines for educational programs to prepare nurses for practice, using fetal heart monitoring techniques. Educational programs include both core and ongoing instruction. A core instructional program includes the essential theoretical and clinical principles to achieve minimal competency. Ongoing instruction includes additional theoretical and clinical education to maintain competency. Nurses are encouraged to refer to institutional policy and related nurse practice acts to determine the scope of nursing practice regarding fetal heart monitoring and antepartum fetal surveillance in individual practice settings.

Antepartum Fetal Surveillance
Nursing practice competencies

Nurses with responsibility for performing antepartum fetal surveillance should demonstrate competency in the application and use of external electronic and auscultatory fetal monitoring equipment and the interpretation of data. Before assuming responsibility for antepartum monitoring, the nurse should be able to do the following:

1. Describe antepartum testing criteria and indications for testing, for example, high-risk pregnancy
2. Provide patient education regarding the procedure and its purpose
3. Prepare the patient; perform complete assessment, including Leopold's maneuvers; palpate the fundus; apply the external electronic fetal monitor
4. Recognize contraindications to the use of oxytocin and nipple stimulation
5. Conduct the prescribed antepartum test
6. Implement interventions per protocol for nonreassuring findings
7. Communicate the content of electronic fetal monitoring data for final interpretation in accordance with institutional policy
8. Document appropriate entries in the written or computerized patient record and the electronic fetal monitor tracing or storage disk
9. Discontinue electronic fetal monitoring according to institutional policy, procedure, and protocol
10. Communicate appropriate follow-up information to the patient

Biophysical profile components, including fetal movement, tone, breathing, and amniotic fluid volume, and other ultrasound assessments, such as fetal position and placental grading and location, may be performed in accordance with institutional policy and the nurse practice act after appropriate educational and clinical instruction in the technique.

Educational guidelines

Three to four hours of didactic instruction specific to antepartum fetal heart monitoring is considered the minimum requirement. Didactic instruction should be followed by supervised clinical experience prior to independent nursing practice. The period of supervised clinical experience required to achieve competency varies with the individual and the practice setting.

Additional didactic instruction and supervised clinical experience specific to antepartum fetal surveillance with ultrasound will vary with the individual and the practice setting.

Didactic content outline

I. Elements of antepartum fetal surveillance
   A. Maternal-fetal physiology
   B. Indication for testing
   C. Methods and interpretation
      1. Nonstress test
      2. Contraction stress test
         (a) Spontaneous
         (b) Nipple stimulation
         (c) Oxytocin
   D. Contraindications for use of oxytocin and nipple stimulation
      1. Ultrasound evaluation, biophysical profile, and other similar noninvasive assessments, according to institutional policy and nurse practice acts
II. Patient education
   A. Indication for testing
   B. Test procedure
   C. Test results
   D. Follow-up
III. Nursing accountability
   A. Policies, procedures, and protocols
   B. Standards of practice
   C. Follow-up: interpretation and reporting protool
   D. Documentation in the written or computerized patient record and on the electronic fetal monitor tracing or storage disk
   E. Legal and ethical issues
   F. Lines of authority and responsibility (chain of command)

Clinical learning experiences and evaluation

The sequence and specific nature of clinical learning experiences can be adapted to accommodate clinical instructors' or preceptors' styles and individual learners' needs.

A. Practice sessions should include a policy, procedure, and protocol manual review and also may include the following:
   1. Electronic fetal monitor tracing review sessions
   2. Small group discussion/case studies
   3. Clinical conferences (multidisciplinary)
   4. Role-play situations
   5. Videotaped observation and follow-up discussion
   6. Computer simulation
   7. One-to-one tutorial
   8. Self-study
B. Practicum
   1. Demonstration with return demonstration of equipment, setup, application, and calibration
   2. Demonstration with return demonstration of equipment maintenance
C. Clinical application of the nursing process under the supervision of the instructor or preceptor
   1. Instruction of the patient and family
   2. Selection of method of assessment
   3. Application of technology (including calibration)
   4. Recognition of technology errors and limitations
   5. Formulation of a nursing diagnosis or nursing problem
   6. Intervention
   7. Documentation in the written or computerized patient record and on the electronic fetal monitor tracing or storage disk
   8. Evaluation and follow-up

Competency validation

Evaluation of didactic and clinical learning validates competency. Evaluation can be ongoing during the learning process or conducted at the conclusion of the learning experiences. The components that comprise competency validation include the following:

A. Written or verbal exercises such as
   1. Examination
   2. Case study analysis
   3. Electronic fetal monitor tracing interpretation sessions
   4. Interpretation of hospital policies, procedures, and protocols
   5. Identification of appropriate lines of authority and respon-

sibility (chain of command)

B. Observation by instructor or preceptor of nurse providing patient care in fetal heart monitoring clinical situations

C. Documentation of competency in the fetal surveillance technique before the nurse functions independently

---

Intrapartum Fetal Heart Monitoring
Nursing practice competencies

To function competently in the use of intrapartum fetal heart monitoring, the nurse should demonstrate competency in the application and use of auscultatory and electronic fetal monitoring equipment and interpretation of data. The intrapartum nurse should therefore be able to do the following:

A. Implement the appropriate fetal heart monitoring method based on patient status, hospital policy, and current standards of practice recommended by professional organizations

B. Explain the principles of the chosen method of fetal heart monitoring to the patient and her support person(s)

C. Identify the limitations of information produced by each method of monitoring

D. Demonstrate competency in fetal heart monitoring by auscultation

 1. Perform complete assessment, including Leopold's maneuvers, to determine fetal position and palpating the fundus to determine appropriate site for auscultation

 2. Apply fetoscope or Doppler device to the appropriate site

 3. Palpate uterine contractions for frequency, duration, and intensity; confirm uterine rest between contractions; determine if abnormal findings are present

 4. Identify and determine the baseline fetal heart rate and rhythm

 5. Identify the presence of fetal heart rate changes with or between uterine contractions

 6. Determine if findings are reassuring or nonreassuring and implement appropriate nursing interventions, including additional fetal monitoring methods

 7. Identify the clinical situations, based on fetal heart monitoring findings, in which immediate notification of the primary health care provider is appropriate

 8. Communicate the findings from auscultation, interpreta-

tion of findings, and resulting nursing intervention(s) in written and verbal form in an appropriate and timely manner

9. Document appropriate entries on the written or computerized patient record

10. Demonstrate appropriate maintenance of auscultation equipment

E. Demonstrate use of electronic fetal monitor

1. Perform complete assessment, including Leopold's maneuvers, palpate the fundus, and auscultate the fetal heart rate prior to application of the transducers

2. Apply external transducers, and adjust the electronic fetal monitor accordingly

3. Prepare the patient, set up the equipment, and complete connections for the fetal electrode with and without intrauterine pressure catheter

4. Calibrate the monitor for the use of the intrauterine pressure catheter

5. Identify technically inadequate tracings, and take appropriate corrective action

6. Obtain and maintain an adequate tracing of the fetal heart and uterine contractions

7. Interpret uterine contraction frequency, duration, intensity, and baseline resting tone as appropriate, based on monitoring method, and determine if abnormal findings are present

8. Identify baseline fetal heart rate and rhythm, variability, and the presence of periodic and nonperiodic changes

9. Determine if findings are reassuring or nonreassuring and implement appropriate nursing interventions

10. Identify the clinical situations, based on fetal heart monitoring findings, in which immediate notification of the primary health care provider is appropriate

11. Communicate the content of electronic fetal monitoring data, interpretation of data, and resulting nursing intervention(s) in written and verbal form in an appropriate and timely manner

12. Document appropriate entries in the written or computerized patient record and on the electronic fetal monitoring tracing or storage disk

13. Demonstrate appropriate maintenance of electronic fetal

monitoring equipment

   14. Demonstrate appropriate storage and retrieval of fetal heart monitoring data

Educational guidelines

The content of educational programs specific to intrapartum fetal heart monitoring should include didactic instruction to meet nursing practice competencies, followed by a period of supervised clinical experience prior to independent nursing practice. The format for presenting didactic instruction may vary, depending on content objectives. A minimum of 8 hours is recommended to cover the core instructional content.

   The period of supervised clinical experience required to achieve competency may vary with the individual. As with the core content, ongoing instructional programs may be adapted as necessary to accommodate instructors' and individual learners' needs.

Didactic content outline

  I. Introduction to fetal heart monitoring
    A. Goals of fetal heart monitoring
      1. Determine fetal heart rate characteristics and uterine activity
      2. Assess fetal well-being
    B. Methods of monitoring
      1. Auscultation and palpation
      2. Electronic fetal monitoring
        (a) Continuous
        (b) Intermittent
      3. Combination of methods
  II. Elements of instrumentation and assessment
    A. Uterine activity monitoring
      1. Palpation
        (a) Principles
        (b) Techniques
        (c) Sources of error and limitations
        (d) Benefits and risks
      2. External electronic: tocodynamometer
        (a) Principles
        (b) Application and care during use
        (c) Sources of error and limitations

            (d) Benefits and risks
        3. Internal electronic: intrauterine pressure catheter
            (a) Types and principles
                (1) Fluid-filled catheters
                (2) Transducer-tipped catheters
            (b) Application and care during use
            (c) Calibration
            (d) Sources of error
            (e) Benefits and risks
    B. Fetal heart rate
        1. External: auscultation
            (a) Types and principles
                (1) Doppler
                (2) Fetoscope
            (b) Techniques
            (c) Sources of error and limitations
            (d) Benefits and risks
        2. External electronic: ultrasound transducer
            (a) Principles of Doppler/ultrasound
            (b) Application and care during use
            (c) Sources of error and limitations
            (d) Benefits and risks
        3. Internal electronic: fetal electrode
            (a) Principles of cardiotachometry
            (b) Application and care during use
            (c) Sources of error and limitations
            (d) Benefits and risks
    C. Equipment maintenance
III. Fetal oxygenation
    A. Physiology of fetal oxygenation
        1. Uteroplacental circulation
        2. Exchange mechanisms
        3. Effects of uterine contractions
        4. Acid-base homeostasis
    B. Pathophysiology of fetal oxygenation
        1. Maternal
            (a) Impaired circulation
            (b) Impaired oxygen exchange
        2. Uterine contraction
            (a) Endogenous causes
            (b) Exogenous causes

       3. Placental
          (a) Impaired circulation
          (b) Impaired oxygen exchange
       4. Umbilical cord
          (a) Compression
          (b) Occlusion
          (c) Compromised perfusion
       5. Fetal
          (a) Impaired circulation
          (b) Impaired oxygen exchange

IV. Interpretation of fetal heart monitoring data
    A. Uterine activity
       1. Resting tone
       2. Contraction frequency
       3. Contraction duration
       4. Contraction intensity
    B. Baseline fetal heart rate and rhythm
       1. Rate and rhythm
          (a) Mechanism (intrinsic and extrinsic control)
             (1) Nervous system control
             (2) Myocardial control
             (3) Endocrine control
             (4) Gestational age influence
          (b) Interpretation
             (1) Normal
             (2) Abnormal
                (a) Tachycardia
                (b) Bradycardia
                (c) Dysrhythmia/Arrhythmia
                (d) Sinusoidal and pseudosinu-
                    soidal*
       2. Variability*: short- and long-term
          (a) Mechanism
          (b) Interpretation
             (1) Reassuring
             (2) Nonreassuring
    C. Periodic fetal heart rate changes*
       1. Accelerations
          (a) Characteristics
          (b) Mechanisms
          (c) Significance

*Electronic fetal monitoring only.

    2. Early decelerations
       (a) Characteristics
       (b) Mechanisms
       (c) Significance
    3. Late decelerations
       (a) Characteristics
       (b) Mechanisms
       (c) Significance
    4. Variable decelerations
       (a) Characteristics
       (b) Mechanisms
       (c) Significance
    5. Prolonged decelerations
       (a) Characteristics
       (b) Mechanisms
       (c) Significance
  D. Nonperiodic fetal heart rate changes*
    1. Accelerations
       (a) Characteristics
       (b) Mechanisms
       (c) Significance
    2. Variable decelerations
       (a) Characteristics
       (b) Mechanisms
       (c) Significance
    3. Prolonged decelerations
       (a) Characteristics
       (b) Mechanisms
       (c) Significance
  E. Auscultated fetal heart changes
    1. Numerical rate
    2. Rhythm
    3. Gradual increase or decrease
    4. Abrupt increase or decrease
V. Nursing process
  A. Assessment
    1. Review of prenatal history
    2. Clinical status of the mother and fetus
    3. Fetal heart rate characteristics and interpretation
    4. Uterine contraction characteristics and interpretation
    5. Documentation

*Electronic fetal monitoring only.

B. Diagnosis
   1. Reassuring
   2. Nonreassuring
C. Planning and intervention
   1. Independent nursing actions
   2. Fetal heart monitoring findings necessitating immediate notification of primary health-care provider
   3. Documentation
   4. Nursing accountability
      (a) Policies, procedures, and protocols
      (b) Standards of practice
      (c) Legal and ethical issues
      (d) Lines of authority and responsibility (chain of command)
D. Evaluation
   1. Response to intervention
   2. Documentation
   3. Continuing plan of nursing care based on response to intervention

Clinical learning experiences and evaluation

The suggested clinical learning experiences and evaluation exercises (p. 158 under "Antepartum Fetal Surveillance") are also appropriate techniques to achieve competency in intrapartum fetal heart monitoring.

Competency validation

The suggested competency validation exercises (p. 159 under "Antepartum Fetal Surveillance") are also appropriate techniques to validate competency in intrapartum fetal heart monitoring.

Summary

This document provides guidelines for educational preparation to achieve competency in fetal heart monitoring. Nurses should participate annually in reviews and clinical update sessions to maintain competency in fetal heart monitoring. Participation in the clinical learning experiences (p. 158) is encouraged. Maintaining the quality of individual practice in accordance with current guidelines and standards is an inherent responsibility of the professional nurse.

Resources

To obtain information on NAACOG resources regarding fetal heart monitoring, call the NAACOG Fulfillment Department at 1-800-673-8499, extension 2464, or from Canada, 1-800-245-0231, extension 2464.

To obtain information on current ACOG resources addressing fetal monitoring and surveillance, contact the ACOG Resource Center at 1-800-673-8499, extension 2518, or from Canada, 1-800-245-0231, extension 2518.

As a benefit of NAACOG membership, you may request a search of the literature on any topic, including fetal surveillance and fetal heart monitoring. Contact the ACOG Resource Center at 1-800-673-8499, extension 2518, or from Canada, 1-800-245-0231, extension 2518.

This publication was developed by a NAACOG ad hoc committee as a resource to OGN nursing. Guidelines are reviewed every 5 years and revised if necessary. These guidelines do not define a standard of care, and they are not intended to dictate exclusive courses of practice. These guidelines present general, recognized recommendations that are intended to provide a foundation and direction for specialty nursing practice. Variations and innovations that demonstrably improve the quality of patient care are to be encouraged rather than restricted. Guidelines do not replace the NAACOG Standards, but rather expand on the principles suggested therein.

Author's note: A NAACOG position statement on *Nursing Responsibilities in Implementing Intrapartum Fetal Heart Rate Monitoring* published in February 1992 and is available from NAACOG.

Task Force Members
Chair

Bonnie Flood Chez, RNC, MSN

Members

Catherine Driscoll, RN, BSN
Judy Schmidt, RNC, EdD

Nursing Practice Competencies and Educational Guidelines Antepartum Fetal Surveillance and Intrapartum Fetal Heart Monitoring has been reviewed by NAACOG members who were designated as nurse consultants. They were selected because of their expertise in fetal surveillance and fetal monitoring. In addition, these guidelines have been reviewed and approved by the NAACOG Committee on Practice. We are indebted to all who shared their time and expertise in the development of this resource.

Appendix B

Protocol for Induction and Augmentation of Labor

Modified from Tucker SM, et al.: Patient care standards: nursing process, diagnosis, and outcome, ed 5, St Louis, 1992, Mosby–Year Book.

Oxytocin Infusion: Augmentation or Induction of Labor

Oxytocin infusion may be used to either begin the labor process or to augment a labor that is progressing slowly because of inadequate uterine activity. Indications for induction include but are not limited to the following:

1. Pregnancy-induced hypertension
2. Premature rupture of membranes
3. Chorioamnionitis
4. Suspected fetal jeopardy as evidenced by biochemical or biophysical indications (e.g., fetal growth retardation, postterm gestation, and isoimmunization)
5. Maternal medical problems (e.g., diabetes mellitus, renal disease, and chronic obstructive pulmonary disease)
6. Fetal demise
7. Postterm gestation

Relative contraindications to inductions include but are not limited to the following:

1. Placenta or vasa previa
2. Nonlongitudinal lie
3. Cord presentation
4. Presenting part above the pelvic inlet
5. Prior classical uterine incision
6. Active genital herpes infection
7. Pelvic structural deformities
8. Invasive cervical carcinoma

Assessment
Observations/Findings

Dysfunctional labor pattern (Table B-1)
Absence of cephalopelvic disproportion
Bishop Score (Table B-2)

Table B-1   Dysfunctional labor patterns

	Nullipara	Multipara
Prolonged latent phase	>21 hr	>14 hr
Protracted active phase	<1.2 cm/hr	<1.5 cm/hr
Secondary arrest: *no change*	>2 hr	>2 hr
Prolonged deceleration phase	>3 hr	>1 hr
Protracted descent	<1 cm/hr	<2 cm/hr
Arrest of descent	>1 hr	>½ hr

Table B-2   Bishop scoring system

	Score			
Area of Assessment	0	1	2	3
Station of presenting part	−3	−2	−1/0	+1/+2
Dilitation in cm	0	1–2	3–4	>5
Effacement in cm	>2.5	2	1	<0.5
Consistency	Firm	Medium	Soft	—
Position of os	Posterior	Central	Anterior	—

Laboratory/Diagnostic studies

FHR-UC monitoring
Cephalopelvic disproportion (CPD) measurements
Ultrasound

Potential complications

Fetal distress
  Hyperactive fetus
  Fetal tachycardia: above 160 bpm
  Fetal bradycardia: below 120 bpm
  Late decelerations
    Prolonged deceleration
  Severe variable decelerations
Uterine hyperstimulation
  Contractions longer than 90 sec
  Contractions occurring more frequently than q2 min (tachy-
    systole)
  Peak pressure of contraction above 90 mm Hg pressure
  Inadequate uterine relaxation: less than 30 sec between con-
    tractions
  Intrauterine resting tone above 15 mm Hg pressure between
    contractions
  Sustained tetanic uterine contraction
Meconium-stained amniotic fluid
Maternal hypertension
Water intoxication
  Rising BP
  Edema of face and fingers and around the eyes
  Shortness of breath
  Difficulty breathing
  Urinary output <30 to 50 ml/hr
Abruptio placentae: sudden, severe uterine pain
Rupture of vasa previa
Precipitate delivery
Hemorrhage
Shock
Uterine rupture
Amniotic fluid embolism

Medical management

Baseline FHR-UC recording
Oxytocin infusion at a rate of 0.5 mU/min and increasing for

desired results at 20- to 60-minute intervals in increments of 1 to 2 mU/min, not to exceed 20 mU/min

Continuous FHR-UC monitoring

Analgesia

Administer

　　Tocolytic agents for excessive uterine activity that persists after oxytocin is discontinued, supportive treatment provided (lateral position and oxygen by mask), and fetal distress is present.

　　Terbutaline 0.25 mg IV push or magnesium sulfate 4 grams, 10% solution over 15 to 20 minutes IV

Nursing diagnoses/Interventions/Evaluation

■ NDX:　Potential for injury related to augmentation of labor related to uterine hyperstimulation

See Care of Mother in First Stage of Labor (Appendix D)

Maintain complete bed rest

Ensure that physician is immediately available

Apply fetal monitoring; obtain baseline strip before starting IV oxytocin

Place patient in comfortable position; lateral position is preferred

Always piggyback oxytocin solution into main IV line close to needle insertion site (10 U oxytocin in 1000 ml IV fluid = 10 mU/ml)

Administer oxytocin via a controlled infusion device as ordered

Monitor dose in mU/min q15 min and before each increase

Increase rate of oxytocic solution as ordered to produce contractions q2 to 3 min of 30 to 60 sec duration

Monitor patency of parenteral system

Check BP, P, and FHR q15 to 30 min or as ordered,

Observe contractions for frequency, duration, strength, and relaxation q5 min for five times, then q15 to 30 min and prn

Administer analgesics as ordered

Assist in breathing and relaxation techniques

Measure intake and output q2h

Prepare for delivery as indicated

Reinforce physician's explanation of reason for augmentation
   or induction of labor
Expected outcome/Evaluation. Mother and fetus are not compromised as a result of oxytocin infusion.

■ NDX: Knowledge deficit regarding lack of information about
          oxytocin infusion procedure

Reinforce physician's explanations
Discuss indications for procedure
Explain methodology of administration
Discuss expected effects of oxytocin induction/augmentation
   of labor
Explain differences between induction/augmentation and nor-
   mal, spontaneous contractions
Expected outcome/Evaluation. Patient and significant other
verbalize understanding of procedure, indications for it, and ex-
pected effects.

Appendix C

Protocol for Management of Preterm Labor

Modified from Tucker SM, et al: Patient care standards: nursing process, diagnosis, and outcome, ed 5, St Louis, 1992, Mosby–Year Book.

Preterm Labor

Physiological process by which the fetus is expelled from the uterus before the completion of the thirty-seventh week of gestation

Assessment

Observations/Findings

Uterine contractions
Every 10 min or less (6 to 8 uterine contraction/hour)
Lasting 30 sec or more
Progressive cervical dilatation: ≥50% effacement or ≥2 cm dilatation
Complaints of back pain or pressure

Laboratory/Diagnostic studies

Electronic fetal monitoring (EFM)
Fetoscope/Doppler
Urinalysis
CBC
Cervical cultures, including group B streptococcus
Amniocentesis to assess fetal lung maturity and presence of infection
Maternal and fetal baseline ECG
Electrolytes
Blood glucose

Potential complications

Compromised infant at birth
- Prematurity
- Small-for-gestational-age infant
- Respiratory distress syndrome

Tocolysis (magnesium sulfate, terbutaline, or ritodrine)

Magnesium sulfate therapy
- Maternal effects
  - Flushing, sense of warmth
  - Headache
  - Dizziness
  - Respiratory depression
  - Hypotension
  - Hyporeflexia
  - Nystagmus
  - Nausea, vomiting
  - Lethargy
  - Pulmonary edema
- Fetal/neonatal effects
  - Decreased muscle tone
  - Respiratory depression
  - Lethargy, drowsiness
  - Lower Apgar scores with prolonged maternal treatment

Terbutaline therapy
- Maternal effects (same as ritodrine)

Ritodrine therapy
- Maternal effects
  - Tachycardia
  - Palpitations
  - Hypotension
  - Arrhythmias
  - Hypokalemia
  - Chest pain
  - Pulmonary edema
  - Tremors
  - Agitation
  - Headache
  - Elevated blood glucose
  - Hyperlipidemia
- Fetal/neonatal effects
  - Fetal distress

Tachycardia
Bradycardia if severe maternal hypotension
Neonatal hypotension
Neonatal hypoglycemia
Neonatal hypocalcemia
Neonatal irritability

Medical management

Bed rest in left lateral position
Continuous EFM and uterine contraction monitoring for a minimum of 1 hr
Home uterine monitoring as indicated by condition, uterine activity, fetal gestational age and maternal compliance with this regimen
Laboratory tests as indicated
Electrolytes
Blood glucose
IV fluids as indicated
Intake and output
Ultrasound for evaluation of placenta, fetal/uterine anomalies, and gestational age confirmation
Glucocorticoids as indicated
Tocolysis as indicated (magnesium sulfate, terbutaline, or ritodrine hydrochloride)
Antibiotics as indicated

Nursing diagnoses/Interventions/Evaluation

■ NDX: Potential for injury to fetus related to potential for pre-term delivery; potential for injury to mother related to tocolysis therapy

Maintain complete bed rest in side-lying position
Administer IV fluids as ordered
Note frequency, duration, and strength of contractions q15 min and prn; monitor uterine activity with tocotransducer (tocodynamometer) if available
Auscultate FHR q15 to 30 min or electronically monitor with ultrasound
Measure intake and output as ordered

Assist with amniocentesis and/or ultrasound if ordered

Administer any other medications, including corticosteroids, in exact dose, time, and route as ordered

Decrease frequency of nursing functions as patient's preterm labor is arrested

Continuous labor

See Care of Mother in First Stage of Labor (Appendix D)

In addition

Prepare for high-risk infant

Notify neonatologist or pediatrician

Have resuscitative equipment ready for use

Plan to have infant's blood crossmatched if less than 32 weeks' gestation

Monitor FHR electronically if possible

Assist physician with fetal blood sampling as indicated

Consider plotting labor dilation and descent on square-ruled graph paper (labor is usually rapid, but a high frequency of abnormal labors occur as well—Friedman curve)

Provide comfort measures before administering minimal doses of analgesics as ordered

Retain placenta for pathology as ordered

Tocolytic therapy

Magnesium sulfate

Maintain patent IV access

Administer 3 to 6 g IV in a 10% solution over 15 to 30 min for initial dose as ordered

Continue and monitor IV infusion titrated according to uterine response and side effects (i.e., 2 g/hr)

Watch for symptoms of toxicity, discontinue, administer oxygen therapy, and notify physician if toxicity occurs

Respiratory depression

Hypotension

Absence of deep tendon reflexes

Keep antidote for magnesium sulfate toxicity (10% calcium gluconate) at bedside

Monitor and decrease dosage after 24 hr or when uterine contractions subside as ordered

Check vital signs and DTRs q30 min to 1 hr

Continue to monitor uterine activity

Monitor intake and output q1h; should be at least 30 ml urine per hour

Auscultate lungs q4h to 8h for presence of fluid

Monitor fetus with EFM as ordered

Check fetal heart rate with vital signs if no EFM is done

Monitor magnesium sulfate levels

Obtain baseline electrolytes and calcium levels by venipuncture

Terbutaline

Parenteral administration

Administer loading dose of 0.25 mg slowly

For continued therapy add 15 mg terbutaline to 250 ml of 5 DW or NS (this will deliver 60 μg/ml)

Give 5 μg/min and increase dose in 5 μg increments q10 minutes until tocolysis is achieved or until 55 μg/min is reached

Oral therapy

Administer first dose before discontinuing parenteral therapy

Dosage 2.5 to 5.0 mg q4h po until 36 weeks' gestation

Ritodrine hydrochloride

Obtain laboratory data as ordered (may include CBC, electrolytes, and glucose)

Place in left lateral position during infusion

Monitor maternal electrocardiogram (ECG) as ordered

Administer ritodrine (usually 50 μg/min) via infusion pump or controller with drug piggybacked into main IV line, being careful not to exceed maximum dosage of 350 μg/min

Monitor rate and dosage and increase by 50 μg/min q10 min based on maternal and fetal responses as ordered

Do not increase dose and/or discontinue ritodrine if patient demonstrates unacceptable side effects; if maternal heart rate exceeds 140 beats/min; if fetal tachycardia of 180 beats/min or greater persists; if systolic blood pressure is <90 mm Hg or more than a 20% decrease; if diastolic BP is <40 mm Hg

Check BP, P, and FHR q10 min while increasing dosage, then q30 min while patient is receiving IV ritodrine maintenance dose

Monitor FHR and uterine contractions continuously if possible

Measure intake and output

Report undesirable side effects, including headache and palpitations, to physician

Continue to maintain IV infusion for 12 hr after arrest of labor, using smallest dose possible to maintain tocolysis

Adjust dosage of tocolytic agent for patients with diurnal patterns of uterine activity

Auscultate lungs q8h to check for fluid overload

Monitor intake and output q1h

Initiate oral therapy 30 min before discontinuing IV therapy as ordered

Decrease frequency of nursing functions as preterm labor is arrested

Expected outcome/Evaluation. Preterm delivery is avoided; there are no maternal complications of tocolysis therapy

■ NDX: Potential situational low self-esteem related to perceptions and expectations of pregnancy and delivery

Encourage patient to verbalize fears and concerns

Note and document
  Minimal eye contact
  Self-defeating statements and/or behaviors
  Overt expressions of guilt or blame
  Negativity or inadequacy in actions or verbal communications
  Demonstrations of anger

Include significant other in discussions

Provide factual information about placement of blame for initiation and continuation of uterine contractions

Provide positive feedback and encouragement to patient for seeking early interventions

Expected outcome/Evaluation. Patient verbalizes positive feelings about self

■ NDX: Pain related to uterine contractions

Use nonpharmacological measures when appropriate
    Positioning
    Muscular relaxation techniques
    Breathing techniques
    Distraction techniques
Eliminate or minimize other factors that could contribute to pain
    Encourage frequent voiding
    Explain all procedures before executing them
    Answer all questions if possible
    Offer choices to allow for control as patient is able
    Keep patient and significant other informed of changes in labor and fetal status
Explain reasons why analgesic agents may not be appropriate
    Effect on fetal heart rate
    Possible masking of contractions
    Combined side effects of tocolytic agents and analgesia
Provide positive reinforcement and touch as appropriate
Plan nursing care to provide rest periods to promote comfort, sleep, and relaxation
Assess and document stress-contributing factors to perception of pain
Assess and document q30 min
    Frequency and length of contractions
    Location of pain
    Intensity and duration of pain
Expected outcome/Evaluation. Patient will verbalize decreasing or more tolerable discomfort

■ NDX: Knowledge deficit related to lack of information about potential premature labor and delivery

Explain arrested labor
Emphasize importance of maintaining bed rest in side-lying position with bathroom privileges as ordered
Emphasize importance of avoiding intercourse, douching, or nipple stimulation, including preparation of breasts for breastfeeding

Teach name of medication, dosage, frequency of administration, purpose, and toxic side effects

Teach or reinforce instructions if patient will be monitored at home with periodic modern transmission of uterine activity

Emphasize importance of having supportive person to perform housekeeping, cooking, and child care tasks

Discuss signs of labor to report to physician

Emphasize importance of follow-up medical care

Discuss development and gestational stage of fetus

Expected outcome/Evaluation. Patient will demonstrate self-care, and patient and significant other will verbalize understanding of preterm labor and purpose of treatment.

Appendix D

Guidelines for Care of the Patient in Labor: First Stage and Second Stage

Modified from Tucker SM, et al.: Patient care standards: nursing process, diagnosis, and outcome, ed 5, St Louis, 1992, Mosby–Year Book.

First Stage of Labor

Early labor dilatation of 0 to 4 cm with mild to moderate irregular contractions

    Active labor dilation of 4 cm with moderate to strong regular contractions q2 min to 5 min

    Transitional labor dilatation of 8 cm to complete dilatation with strong contractions

Assessment

Observations/Findings

Behavior
- Surge of energy and activity
- Talking frequently
- Anxious
- Fear of isolation

Rupture of membranes

Uterine contractions: regular with increasing intensity and frequency

Transitional labor
- Nausea and vomiting
- Irritability
- Loss of coping mechanism
- Hiccups and/or belching
- Trembling and/or shaking of legs
- Chilling
- Perspiration

Rectal pressure
Urge to push
Hypersensitive abdomen

Laboratory/Diagnostic studies

Baseline laboratory tests
CBC with differential
Blood type, Rh, Indirect Coombs
VDRL serology
Chemistries
Rubella Titer
Hepatitis screen
Varicella Titer
Urinalysis
Cultures as indicated by history of signs and symptoms
Ultrasound/x-ray examination as indicated
Acid-base monitoring

Potential complications

Nonreassuring findings
    Fetal tachycardia: above 160 bpm
    Fetal bradycardia: below 120 bpm
    Meconium-stained amniotic fluid
    Foul-smelling amniotic fluid
Fetal hyperactivity
Monitored labor
    Severe variable decelerations: <70 bpm for more than 30
        sec
    Uncorrectable, repetitive late decelerations of any magnitude
    Absence of variability
    Prolonged deceleration
    Unstable FHR; sinusoidal pattern
Supine hypotension syndrome
Inadequate uterine relaxation
    Contractions lasting longer than 90 sec
    Relaxation between contractions less than 30 sec
Arrest of labor
Amnionitis secondary to prolonged rupture of membranes
Elevated temperature
Distended bladder

Dehydration
Hemorrhage
Prolapsed umbilical cord
Abruptio placentae

Medical management

Laboratory tests as indicated
IV fluids as indicated
Prenatal chart and previous medical chart ordered to labor and
    delivery unit
Vital sign monitoring according to facility policy
Analgesia as indicated
Preparation for selected/indicated anesthesia by anesthesiolo-
    gist/nurse anesthetist
Fetal heart rate-uterine contraction (FHR-UC) monitoring

Nursing diagnoses/Interventions/Evaluation

■ NDX: Potential for injury to mother related to physiological
          processes of labor and to infection secondary to con-
          tamination

Check temperature q2h after rupture of membranes
Consider plotting cervical dilation and fetal descent over time
    on square-ruled graph paper (Friedman curve)
Give enema in early labor if ordered
Administer clear liquids as ordered
Monitor intake and output
Have patient void q2h and prn
Check urine for glucose and protein
Maintain complete bed rest in position of comfort if mem-
    branes are ruptured, especially if presenting part is not yet
    engaged; otherwise, patient may ambulate as tolerated
    Allow patient up to bathroom as ordered if presenting part
        is well applied to cervix
Initiate lactated Ringer's solution or other IV solution as or-
    dered
Prehydrate with 500 to 1000 ml of fluid before anesthetic pro-
    cedure as ordered
Maintain dosing of prelabor medications or drugs as ordered
    (i.e., anticonvulsants, antihypertensives, or methadone)

Expected outcome/Evaluation. Patient does not experience any injury related to labor as evidenced by adequate hydration, skin turgor, voiding pattern (absence of distended bladder)

There is no fever or other evidence of infection

■ NDX: Pain and anxiety related to intensity of uterine contractions and fear of the unknown

Active labor

Give back rub qh and prn between contractions

Apply pressure to sacrum as needed prn during contractions

Explain all procedures

Apply cool compress to forehead prn

Change pad under buttocks when moist q30 min to 60 min and prn

Assist with breathing techniques and teach significant other to assist patient

Change gown and linen as necessary

Turn off bright overhead lights when not needed

Clip call bell to bottom sheet within easy reach to ensure that staff is promptly notified of patient's needs

Relieve discomfort with medication as ordered

Assist physician with local or regional anesthetic; take BP and P q10 min for three times after anesthetic and until stabilized

Avoid talking to patient during contractions

Reposition patient q30 min and prn; lateral position is preferred

Transitional phase of labor

Encourage deep ventilation before and after each contraction when patient is in active labor and during transition period

Avoid urge to push by panting and/or blowing in rapid sequence with contractions until completely dilated

Have emesis basin readily available

Have patient void to ensure empty bladder

Cover feet with blanket or have patient wear socks if chilling occurs

Tell patient that the transition stage usually lasts no more than

1 to 2 hr and then she will be allowed to push and deliver infant

Palpate abdomen very lightly and only as often as necessary if abdomen is hypersensitive

Avoid having persons in labor room who are not directly caring for patient

Accept aggression or other coping behaviors; avoid negative comments

Avoid unnecessary talking or expression of feelings to meet own needs

Focus on patient and support her
   Calm voice
   Touch
   Positive reinforcement after contractions

Expected outcome/Evaluation.   Patient experiences manageable pain and minimal anxiety as evidenced by verbalization of same

Complies with assistive directions by staff

Has continuing positive interaction with significant other/family

■ NDX: Altered oral mucous membrane related to mouth breathing

Administer oral hygiene qh and prn between contractions

Suck on ice chips, wet washcloths, or sour lollipops unless contraindicated

Rinse mouth with water and/or mouthwash

Apply petroleum jelly or antichapping lipsticks to dry lips prn

Expected outcome/Evaluation.   Patient does not experience disruption in tissue layers of oral cavity

■ NDX: Potential for injury to fetus related to uterine contractions of labor and/or uteroplacental insufficiency

Note frequency, duration, and strength of contractions q30 min to 60 min and prn in early labor; increase to q15 min to 30 min in active labor

Auscultate FHR immediately after uterine contractions, preferably for one full minute if not electronically monitored in first stage of labor (q15 min to 30 min and prn)

Check BP and P qh and prn

Check T, P, and R q2h to 4h and prn

Auscultate FHR immediately after membranes rupture or amniotomy is done

Turn mother to left-lateral position, increase rate of plain IV, administer 100% oxygen by face mask, and notify physician immediately if fetal distress is evident by auscultation or electronic fetal monitoring

Expected outcome/Evaluation. Patient delivers an infant in good condition at birth with Apgar score ≥8 at 5 min of age

■ **NDX:**   Anxiety related to lack of knowledge and uncertainty about what to expect during labor

Allay anxiety as much as possible by doing the following:

Explain reasons for performing all procedures

Encourage spouse or significant other to remain with the patient to provide support during labor

Let spouse or significant other listen to fetal heart tones with stethoscope, fetoscope, or ultrasound stethoscope

Provide supportive care based on patient's knowledge of the labor process

Inform waiting family members and friends of patient's progress, and let the patient know that they are interested in her

Reduce environmental stimuli that may contribute to anxiety and tension; provide a relaxed, restful atmosphere

At appropriate intervals reassure the patient that labor is progressing and that both patient and infant are doing fine

Instruct spouse or significant other when and where to change into scrub suit, cap, and mask to be ready to go into delivery room

Expected outcome/Evaluation. Patient verbalizes understanding of process of labor and rationale for procedures

Is supported by significant other in coping with anxiety

Procedural Care of The Patient During the Second Stage of Labor

The stage of expulsion of the fetus, placenta, and membranes from the mother at birth after complete dilatation of the cervix

Assessment
Observations/Findings

Involuntary bearing down
Pushing
Grunting sounds
Extreme anxiety
Vomiting episode
Involuntary shaking of legs
Perspiration between nose and upper lip
Increase in bloody show
Patient stating, "Baby is coming"
Desire to defecate, fear of "making a mess"
Prolonged second stage
    More than 1 hr for multigravidas
    More than 2 hr for primigravidas

Laboratory/Diagnostic studies

Electronic fetal monitoring
Cord blood: gases, pH, and other tests as ordered

Potential complications/Risks

High-risk delivery
Placenta abruptio
Difficult delivery
    Shoulder dystocia
    Breech presentation
    Cephalopelvic disproportion
Forceps delivery
Vacuum extraction
Cesarean section
Infant bruising, fractures

Nursing procedures
Care during delivery

Auscultate FHR q5 min and/or after each push if electronic
    monitor is not used (if electronic monitor was used contin-
    uously during labor, then it should be continued in the de-
    livery room until the time of delivery)
Check BP and P q10 min and prn
Pad stirrups

Administer oxygen by mask at 10 to 12 L/min as ordered

Understand that low- to semi-Fowler's position with lateral tilt is prefereed while pushing

Assist with breathing techniques

Deep ventilation before and after each contraction

Breathing technique and pushing with contractions

Observe perineum while pushing

Notify physician if second stage is prolonged

Prepare perineum according to hospital procedure

Place nurse, spouse, and/or labor coach at head of delivery table to encourage patient during delivery process

Encourage long, sustained pushing rather than frequent short pushes

Encourage complete relaxation between contractions

Reassure patient that she is doing well and is advancing the infant with each push

Apply cool moist cloth to forehead as needed

Have DeLee suction catheter available and ready to use if meconium-stained amniotic fluid is present

Plan for suctioning of naso-oropharynx after delivery of fetal head and before delivery of thorax to prevent meconium aspiration

Assist physician or nurse-midwife as needed

Immediate postdelivery care

Permit mother to inspect infant as soon as possible

Place infant on maternal abdomen to provide skin-to-skin contact if delivery room is warm

Defer neonatal eye therapy for 1 to 2 hr after birth to promote eye contact with mother

Check BP and P q10 min to 15 min for four times and prn

Add oxytocic drug as ordered to parenteral fluids

Palpate fundus, noting location and tonus q5 min to 10 min for four times

Administer perineal care before removing legs from stirrups

Place sterile perineal pad and/or pad under buttocks before transporting patient to recovery area

Place ice pack on episiotomy unless otherwise ordered

Assist with infant's warm water bath as indicated if infant's temperature is stable

Maintain mother's warmth with blankets as needed

Place radiant heat warmer over upper part of mother's bed or place dry, warmly blanketed infant next to mother so that she can visually inspect, touch, and/or breastfeed nude infant while preventing neonatal heat loss

Let mother and spouse and/or labor coach be with infant in delivery area, providing them with as much privacy as feasible unless this is contraindicated by maternal or fetal condition

Encourage mother to freely express her feelings about herself and her infant

Explain that behaviors manifested in labor are normal and there is no reason to apologize if mother is apologetic for behavior while in labor

Appendix E

Selected Pattern Interpretation

Fetal Tachycardia

SIGNAL SOURCE	Spiral electrode and tocotransducer
FHR	Baseline: 190 to 200 bpm
	Variability: Average
	Periodic changes: No significant changes; a mild variable deceleration occurs in panel 30266.
UTERINE ACTIVITY	Frequency: 2 to 2½ minutes
	Duration: 30 to 40 seconds

Note the wide excursion vertical lines, probably caused by electrical "noise" or interference. If these lines were more frequent and consistent, they would suggest a fetal dysrhythmia.

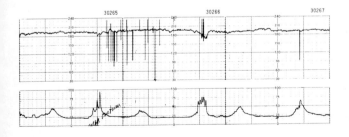

Fetal Bradycardia

SIGNAL SOURCE	Spiral electrode and intrauterine catheter
FHR	Baseline: 110 bpm
	Variability: Average
	Periodic changes: No significant changes
UTERINE ACTIVITY	Frequency: 3 to 3½ minutes
	Duration: 50 to 60 seconds
	Intensity: 50 to 65 mm Hg
	Resting tone: 5 mm Hg

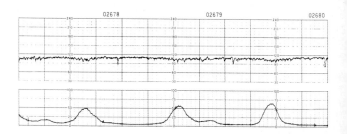

Flat Baseline

SIGNAL SOURCE	Spiral electrode and tocotransducer
FHR	Baseline: 140 to 150 bpm
	Variability: Minimal
	Periodic changes: No significant changes

This fetus was 3 weeks overdue and later delivered spontaneously with a meconium-stained placenta, birth weight of 4067 g (9 lb 1¼ oz), and Apgar scores of 4 at 1 minute and 7 at 5 minutes of age.

UTERINE ACTIVITY	Contractions are either not present, or the tocotransducer is misplaced. The uterine activity demonstrated here is normal for the patient who is not in labor. Respiratory movements are clearly seen.

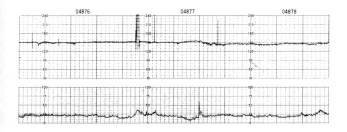

Acceleration of FHR with UC

SIGNAL SOURCE   Spiral electrode and tocotransducer

FHR   Baseline: 140 to 150 bpm

                     Variability: Average

                     Periodic changes: Acceleration of FHR
                     occurs with each contraction. The ampli-
                     tude of the acceleration is markedly in-
                     creased when the patient pushes with
                     contractions.

UTERINE ACTIVITY   Frequency: 2½ minutes

                     Duration: 40 to 50 seconds

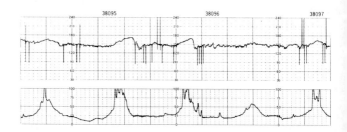

Acceleration of FHR with UC

SIGNAL SOURCE	Spiral electrode and intrauterine catheter
FHR	Baseline: 130 bpm
	Variability: Average

Periodic changes: Acceleration of fetal heart rate occurs with each contraction and with fetal movement as evidenced by the spikes in the UA panel just before the two middle contractions. Sometimes acceleration of FHR with contractions or before contractions makes the FHR look as if late decelerations are occurring, when given a casual glance. Therefore it is important to identify the baseline rate and note the timing of the acceleration or deceleration in relation to the uterine contraction.

UTERINE ACTIVITY   Frequency: 3 to 3½ minutes

Duration: 60 to 70 seconds

Intensity: Probably 75 to 85 mm Hg

Resting tone: Probably 30 to 35 mm Hg

The strain gauge has not been opened to room air and calibrated. The resting tone and intensity of the contractions are most likely much lower than are reflected in this tracing.

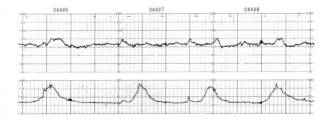

Early Decelerations

SIGNAL SOURCE   Ultrasound and tocotransducer

FHR   Baseline: 120 bpm

Variability: Not specific with ultrasound but probably minimal

Periodic changes: Consistent early decelerations occur with each contraction because of head compression.

UTERINE ACTIVITY   Frequency: 2 to 3 minutes

Duration: 40 to 50 seconds

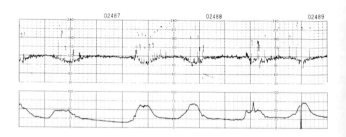

Mild Variable Decelerations

SIGNAL SOURCE	Spiral electrode and tocotransducer
FHR	Baseline: 140 bpm
	Variability: Average
	Periodic changes: Mild variable decelerations in FHR occur with each contraction. This frequently occurs with pushing and signals the second stage of labor.
UTERINE ACTIVITY	Frequency: 1½ to 2 minutes
	Duration: 30 to 40 seconds

Spikes of uterine pressure above 50 mm Hg indicate maternal pushing.

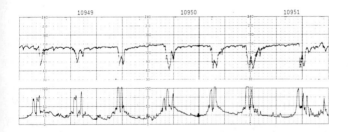

Fetal Cardiac Arrhythmia

SIGNAL SOURCE Spiral electrode and intrauterine catheter

FHR Baseline: 170 bpm; the vertical excursions from the baseline indicate a cardiac arrhythmia. If they were less frequent and more random, they would suggest electrical interference or "noise." Clinically, this pattern is not a cause for consideration of termination of labor. Most fetal cardiac arrhythmias disappear after birth and are not considered a sign of fetal distress.

Variability: Minimal

UTERINE ACTIVITY Frequency: 1½ to 6 minutes

Duration: 50 to 60 seconds

Intensity: 50+ mm Hg with patient pushing

Resting tone: 10 mm Hg

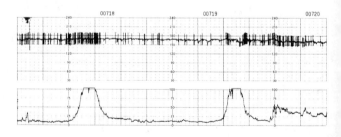

External Mode of Monitoring—Clear Tracing

SIGNAL SOURCE	Ultrasound and tocotransducer
FHR	Baseline: 140 bpm
	Variability: Not specific with ultrasound but probably average
	Periodic changes: No significant changes
UTERINE ACTIVITY	Frequency: 2 to 2½ minutes
	Duration: 30 to 50 seconds

Note the zigzag respiratory movements of the uterine activity panel.

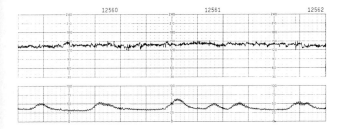

Loose Spiral Electrode with Complete Cervical Dilatation

SIGNAL SOURCE   Spiral electrode and tocotransducer

FHR   Baseline: 136 bpm in panel 55986. The
                     sudden loss of FHR signal in panel
                     55987 is due to loose spiral electrode
                     (lead) since complete dilatation has oc-
                     curred. The actual FHR was then auscul-
                     tated at 136 bpm, which is consistent
                     with the previously known baseline.

                     Variability: Unable to determine

                     Periodic changes: Unable to determine

UTERINE ACTIVITY   Frequency: 2½ to 3 minutes

                     Duration: 50 to 90 seconds

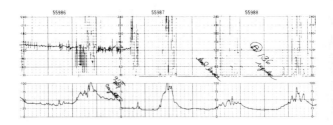

Coupling of Uterine Contractions

SIGNAL SOURCE	Spiral electrode and intrauterine catheter
FHR	Baseline: 130 bpm
	Variability: Average
	Periodic changes: No significant changes
UTERINE ACTIVITY	Frequency: 1½ to 4½ minutes
	Duration: 40 seconds
	Intensity: 60 mm Hg
	Resting tone: 5 mm Hg

Laboring patterns vary among individuals. Note the characteristic coupling of uterine contractions in this tracing.

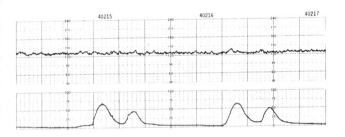

Bibliography

American Academy of Pediatrics and American College of Obstetricians and Gynecologists: Guidelines for perinatal care. Washington, DC, 1988, AAP/ACOG.

ACOG: Antepartum fetal surveillance, Technical Bulletin No 107, Washington, DC, August 1987, American College of Obstetricians and Gynecologists.

ACOG: Assessment of fetal and newborn acid-base status, Technical Bulletin No 127, Washington, DC, April 1989, American College of Obstetricians and Gynecologists.

American College of Obstetricians and Gynecologists: *Intrapartum* fetal heart rate monitoring, ACOG Technical Bulletin No 132, Washington, DC, September 1989, American College of Obstetricians and Gynecologists.

Afriat CI: Electronic fetal monitoring, Rockville, Md, 1989, Aspen Publishers.

Auyeung RM, Goldkrand JW: Vibroacoustic stimulation and nursing intervention in the nonstress test, *JOGN* 20(3):232-238, 1991.

Banta HD, Thacker SB: Costs and benefits of electronic fetal monitoring: a review of the literature, National Center for Health Services Research: Research Report Series, US Department of Health, Education and Welfare, April 1979, DHEW Publication No (PHS) 79-3245.

Benson RC, et al.: Fetal heart rate as a predictor of fetal distress: a report from the Collaborative Project, *Obstet Gynecol* 32:529, 1968.

Capeless EL, Mann LI: Use of breast stimulation for antepartum stress testing, *Obstet Gynecol* 64(5):641-645, 1984.

Clark SL: Do we still need fetal scalp blood sampling? *Contemp Ob/Gyn* 33(3):75-86, 1989.

Clark SL: How a modified NST improves fetal surveillance, *Contemp Ob/Gyn* 35(5):45-48, 1990.

Clark S, Gimovsky M, and Miller F: The scalp stimulation test: a clinical alternative to fetal scalp pH blood sampling, *Am J Obstet Gynecol* 148:274, 1984.

Clark S, Sabey P, and Jolley K: Nonstress testing with acoustic stimulation and amniotic volume assessment: 5973 tests without unexpected fetal death, *Am J Obstet Gynecol* 160:694, 1989.

Dehaan J and others: Quantitative evaluation of the fixed heart rate during pregnancy and labor, *Eur J Obstet Gynecol* 3:103, 1971.

Dicker D and others: Effect of intracranial pressure changes on the fetal heart rate: study of a hydrocephalic fetus, *Israel J Med Sci* 19:364, 1983.

Didolkar S, Mutch M: Major/multiple congenital anomalies and intrapartum fetal heart rate pattern, *South Dakota J Med* 39:5, 1979.

Freeman RK, Garite TJ, and Nageotte MP: *Fetal heart rate monitoring,* Baltimore, 1991, Williams & Wilkins.

Gaffney SE, Salinger L, and Vintzileos AM: The biophysical profile for fetal surveillance, *MCN* 15(6):356-360, 1990.

Gilstrap LC, et al.: Diagnosis of birth asphyxia on the basis of fetal pH, Apgar score, and newborn cerebral dysfunction, *Am J Obstet Gynecol* 161:825, 1989.

Hankins GDV: Apgar scores: are they enough? *Contemp Ob/Gyn: Ob-Gyn Law Special Issue* 36:13-25, 1991.

Harvey CJ: Fetal scalp stimulation: enhancing the interpretation of fetal monitor tracings, *J Perinat Neonatal Nurs* 1(1):13-21, 1987.

Haverkamp AD, et al.: A controlled trial of the differential effects of intrapartum fetal monitoring, *Am J Obstet Gynecol* 134(4):399-412, 1979.

Haverkamp AD, et al.: The evaluation of continuous fetal heart rate monitoring in high risk pregnancy, *Am J Obstet Gynecol* 123:310, 1976.

Hon Edward H: An introduction to fetal heart rate monitoring, Wallingford, Conn, 1975 (Distributed by Corometrics).

Huddleston JF: Contraction stress test by intermittent nipple stimulation, *Obstet Gynecol* 63(5):669-673, 1984.

Jarvis SN, Holloway JS, and Hey EN: Increase in cerebral palsy in normal birth weight babies, *Arch Dis Child* 60:1113, 1985.

Kelso IM, et al.: An assessment of continuous fetal heart rate monitoring in labor: a randomized trial, *Am J Obstet Gynecol* 131:526, 1978.

Leveno KJ, et al.: A prospective comparison of selective and universal electronic fetal monitoring in 34,995 pregnancies, *N Engl J Med* 315:615, 1986.

Luthy DA, et al.: A randomized trial of electronic fetal monitoring in preterm labor, *Obstet Gynecol* 69(5):687-695, 1987.

Manning FA, et al.: Fetal biophysical profile scoring: a prospective study in 1184 high-risk patients, *Am J Obstet Gynecol* 140(3):289-294, 1981.

Manning RA, et al.: Fetal biophysical profile scoring: selective use of the nonstress test, *Am J Obstet Gynecol* 156(3):709-712, 1987.

McDonald D, et al.: The Dublin randomized control trial of intrapartum fetal heart rate monitoring, *Am J Obstet Gynecol* 152:524, 1985.

Menticoglou S, et al.: Severe fetal brain injury without intrapartum asphyxia or trauma, *Obstet Gynecol* 74:457, 1989.

Miyasaki FS, Nevarez F: Saline amnioinfusion for relief of repetitive variable decelerations: a prospective randomized study, *Am J Obstet Gynecol* 153(3):301-306, 1985.

Miyasaki FS, Taylor NA: Saline amnioinfusion for relief of variable or prolonged decelerations, *Am J Obstet Gynecol* 146(6):670-678, 1983.

NAACOG: Fetal heart rate auscultation, OGN Nursing Practice Resource, Washington, DC, March 1990, NAACOG: The Organization for Obstetric, Gynecologic and Neonatal Nurses.

NAACOG: Standards for obstetric, gynecologic, and neonatal nursing, ed 4, Washington, DC, 1991, NAACOG.

NAACOG: Statement: nursing responsibilities in implementing intrapartum fetal heart rate monitoring, Washington, DC, 1989, NAACOG.

Nelson KB, Ellenberg JH: Antecedents of cerebral palsy: multivariate analysis of risk, *N Engl J Med* 315:81, 1986.

Niswander KR: Does substandard obstetric care cause cerebral palsy? *Contemp Ob/Gyn* 30(4):42-60, 1987.

Niswander KR: EFM and brain damage in term and post-term infants, *Contemp Ob/Gyn: Ob/Gyn Law Special Issue* 36:39-50, 1991.

Nocon JJ: Risk management and neurologically impaired infants, *Contemp Ob/Gyn* 36 (Special Issue) 61-68, February 15, 1991.

Obstetric Advisory Committee: Prenatal and intrapartum protocols, Los Angeles, 1991, Perinatal Advisory Council of Los Angeles Communities.

Ombelet W, VanDerMerwe J: Sinusoidal fetal heart rate pattern associated with congenital hydrocephalus, *S Afr Med J* 67:423, 1985.

Page FO, et al.: Correlation of neonatal acid-base status with Apgar scores and fetal heart rate tracings, *Am J Obstet Gynecol* 154(6):1306-1310, 1986.

Parer JT: Handbook of fetal heart rate monitoring, Philadelphia, 1983, WB Saunders.

Platt LD: Predicting fetal health with the biophysical profile, *Contemp Ob/Gyn* 33(2):105-119, 1989.

Rabello YA, Lapidus MR: Fundamentals of electronic fetal monitoring, Wallingford, Conn, 1991, Corometric Medical Systems.

Renou P, et al.: Controlled trial of fetal intensive care, *Am J Obstet Gynecol* 126:470, 1976.

Saling E, Schneider D: Biochemical supervision of the foetus during labour, *J Obstet Gynecol Br Commonwealth* 74:749, 1967.

Shields J, Schifrin B: Perinatal antecedents of CP, *Obstet Gynecol* 71:899, 1988.

Shy KK, Larson EB, and Luthy DA: Evaluating a new technology: the effectiveness of electronic fetal heart rate monitoring, *Annu Rev Public Health* 8:165-190, 1987.

Sleutel MR: An overview of vibrocoustic stimulation, *JOGN* 18(6):447-452, November/December 1989.

Smith CV, et al.: Fetal acoustic stimulation testing: a retrospective experience with fetal acoustic stimulation test, *Am J Obstet Gynecol* 153:567-568, 1985.

Smith CV, Phelan JP, Platt LK, Broussard P, and Paul RH: Fetal acoustic stimulation testing: a randomized clinical comparison with the nonstress test, *Am J Obstet Gynecol* 155(1):131-134, 1986.

Thorp JA, et al.: Routine umbilical cord blood gas determinations? *Am J Obstet Gynecol* 161:600, 1989.

Tucker SM, et al.: Patient care standards: nursing process, diagnosis, and outcome, ed 5, St Louis, 1992, Mosby–Year Book.

VanderMoer P, Gerretsen G, Visser G: Fixed fetal heart rate pattern after intrauterine accidental decerebration, *Obstet Gynecol* 65:125, 1985.

Vintzileos AM, et al.: The use and misuse of the fetal biophysical profile, *Am J Obstet Gynecol* 156(3):527-533, 1987.

Williams RL, Hawes WE: Cesarean section, fetal monitoring and perinatal mortality in California, *Am J Public Health* 69:864, 1979.

Wood C, et al.: A controlled trial of fetal heart rate monitoring in a low-risk population, *Am J Obstet Gynecol* 141:527, 1981.

Index